SENSATIONAL SLIMMING SECRETS

A Revolutionary Pathway To A Healthier
& Slimmer You

RINO SORIANO

Rino Soriano

DISCLAIMER

This book is designed to provide information on holistic health living. It is distributed with the understanding that the author and publisher are not engaged in rendering medical advice or medical claims about your health and well-being. Rino is not a licensed health practitioner or doctor. He is an educator in holistic health and has experience in holistic nutrition, fitness, and supplemental health programs.

Every effort has been made to make this manual complete and as accurate as possible. However, there may be errors in both typographical and content. Therefore, this text should be used as a general guide and not the ultimate source for improving your health. Furthermore, this manual contains holistic health information that is current only up to the printing date.

The main intent of this manual is to educate and entertain. BodyBrilliance LLC and the author Rino Soriano and publisher Flying Hawk Productions shall have neither liability nor responsibility to any person or entity with respect to any loss or damage caused by or allegedly to have been caused, directly or indirectly, by the information in this book.

TABLE OF CONTENTS

PREFACE

Hi there my friend, are you finally ready for the solution to your weight issues? Do you want clarification as why almost every health program or product you have used has not helped you and the millions of overweight people in this world? Will you like to have health simplified to such a degree that you can easily get the results you have been seeking? You really want to know how to do this, yes? Well, what I am about to reveal to you shall knock you outside the galaxy.

You see, most of the information out there about weight reduction is not going to help you get results. I am quite sure that you have tried the diets, the fancy machines, and other so-called weight reduction remedies and you haven't gotten the results you have wanted.

Or, you may have actually gained weight by following such erroneous and untrue paradigms. You have obviously proven to yourself as have millions of other people that these so called weight reduction remedies are not the solution. I live by a simple saying and that is ....**The Proof Is In The Pudding**.

If these so-called weight reduction remedies work as claimed then there would be millions of slim, healthy and happy people.

The Truth is the opposite because we have millions of people who are overweight and even children who are obese now. These people have followed the information that is out there in society and have not gotten lasting results. Therefore, you know by now that information is not going to help you.

For you to get the results you desire you require factual information that is based on sound holistic health principles and validate themselves. If you are ready to finally have the solution to your weight issues, it is here in this book that you shall discover the missing components that you have been waiting for. My intention is to provide you the True solution that you can use to help transform your life.

So, hang onto your hat because you are in for one amazing journey. The information I will present to you throughout this book is the roadmap that you and millions of people have been praying for. I am quite confident that if you follow most or all of what I am setting before you, that your life is going to change in quantum leaps.

In fact, you will be experiencing a whole lot more than just holistic slimming results. You will actually have a roadmap to your evolution and for experiencing your Higher Potentials.

I honestly want you to have the solution you have been looking for. Just be aware that I am not going to hype things up and try to embellish what results you may experience. You shall experience the results that you will allow. You see, the question is not can you get the results you seek, it is how far do you want to take it? How much weight do you want shed? How much fat do you want to vaporize off your body? It can be done in a safe and holistic manner as I teach. I coach people one on one and teach them sound holistic health practices for melting the fat and keeping it off.

Actually, once you learn what I teach, you shall never have to worry about weight issues again. However, like I said, it is up to you the results you experience and how far do you want to go? How much weight do you want to shed off your body and what do you want your body to look like? I can help you do that, you just have to be willing to walk the path.

I have created a simplistic holistic pathway for most people to getting in shape, vaporizing the fat and even getting rid of cellulite. There is a common thread that applies to all these conditions and as I shall teach you in this book, once you know the Truth you will have new eyes to see and a new perspective about your health. Actually, the solution is so simple that you have missed it.

You have missed the solution because what is being taught out there is actually counterproductive and makes people more overweight. In the past 15 years, especially in the US, more and more people have become overweight overall, even though they have followed the weight reduction diets, the cardio programs and the whole list of so called weight reduction remedies.

You see this, right? That more people have become overweight yet they have followed the so called weight reduction solutions. These so called weight reduction solutions have actually contributed to more people experiencing low level health and the gaining of excess weight. Once you learn the simple science of what I am going to teach you, you will see why.

My recommendation to you is to let go of all the beliefs about weight reduction and what you think is True. In order for you to get the results you seek, you must first detox your mind of all the theories that society has brainwashed you with. You then go about learning Truthful information that validates itself. **Truth validates itself every single time. It is a boat that floats.**

So, what I shall teach you validates itself because you go out in your life and see the Truth. I am not here to teach you my theory, I am here to teach you holistic health principles that prove themselves over and over again. Because, once you know how the body functions and what it requires to be at optimal levels then the rest becomes quite simple.

So, if you are ready to shed all the illusions about weight reduction and health for that matter, you are about to embark on one amazing journey my friend. You see, what I am going to teach you here in this book will catapult you to Higher levels of health and well-being. Again, it is because you will be following information and a lifestyle that is conducive to getting results. If you are ready to embark on this amazing journey then let us proceed, shall we?

I shall present to you some of what I call erroneous myths of life that actually appear to be factual on the surface yet they do not validate themselves when you attempt to prove their substance. This information is being posed as the Truth when in fact it is mainly the cause of why more and more people are becoming overweight, obese and out of shape.

Be careful of what you believe because your beliefs may actually cause you to remain overweight and experience low level health. In order for you to experience the results you seek, you must be open minded and learn to discern information that is erroneous and which is True.

I teach principles and practices that validate themselves as they are based on natural laws and simple science of how things function. You require learning how your body functions and what it requires to be at optimum health levels. You also require learning about sound holistic nutrition principles that promote awesome health and well-being. Nutrition is the foundation to your health so it is wise for you to take some time to learn about your body and what it requires to function optimally, don't you think?

You ensure that your car receives the proper octane gas, right? You change the oil and lube it up and get it serviced at the appropriate time, yes? You wash and wax your car and take care of it, right? Well, your body requires care as well, in fact, your body requires a whole lot more than just some care. It requires love, nourishment and cleansing and you are the only one that can provide this you see. How is it that people have been treating their bodies as a machine and their car as they should their body??? Many people treat their cars way better than their body.

Many people know more about how their computers and cell phones work than they do their own body? Wouldn't you say that this is not healthy or wise? Wouldn't it make sense to learn about your body and what it requires to function optimally and how to maintain High levels of health and well-being?

I am here to remind you that your body is a Sacred Temple and it is your vehicle for experiencing this game called life. It is your duty to take care of your vehicle as best you can. My main message to you is invest in your health and do everything you can to be as healthy as possible because this shall translate into you being the person you are meant to be.

How can you go out in life and contribute in a positive way if you have low level health and are overweight and obese? You can't do it my friend. To be your Highest Potential Self and live your Highest Life, you require being optimally healthy so that you may express your talents and gifts to the world.

You do not help yourself or anyone by being out of shape, overweight, obese or have low level health. Please, for your sake and the sake of humanity, make the decision to begin your path to wellness and your healing.

You can do it, I know you can. This is why I offer my services to people, because I know most people have been through quite a bunch and are looking for the True solution to their weight issues. I also know that most of the information being taught out there is not going to get you lasting results. Like I said, that information will lead you to become more overweight and more frustrated. I have a great comprehension of how to help people get the weight off and have it last.

So, the path is here if you choose? The decision must come from you if you want to walk it. I offer my coaching programs to people like you because I want you to experience happiness and feel good inside. I want you to be healthy and fit and radiant.

By you being healthy you then can help others by being an example of what is possible. You shall be a shining example of a healthy, fit and radiant person. This starts today with a choice, your choice to walk the holistic pathway to optimum health and a slimmer you. Are you ready?

CHAPTER 1

WHY YOU ARE OVERWEIGHT

I am now going to teach you about holistic health, holistic nutrition and what your body requires to function optimally. You see, just because you fill your belly does not mean that you are nourishing your body and cells. In fact, the way most people and you are going at nutrition is way off balance and this actually degenerates your body and sets you up for weight gain.

Most of the foods at the grocery stores are not foods that nourish your body. In fact, they are one of the main causes of why so many people are overweight. These grocery store foods are devoid of nutrition and they also contain preservatives, binders and fillers that are toxic to your system.

Here are some facts for you just in case you are not up to par on what the Truth is about the produce and food products in grocery stores. First, is that most of the produce being grown on farms is devoid of vital nutrition due to the soils being deficient in viable bio-nutrients that your body requires to function optimally. You see, the soil is supposed to contain hundreds of vital bio-nutrients necessary for you to be healthy.

What most people are not aware of is that the common farming practices have actually wiped out the healthy micro-bacteria and fungi that are the main creators of the hundreds of vital bio-nutrients that your body requires on a daily basis.

The modern way of farming is not healthy and has literally removed the main producers of the vital nutrients that are supposed to be in healthy soil. This is a Divine process that has been disrupted by conventional practices and has many consequences, one being that your body will not receive its daily supply of life giving nutrients.

When your body does not receive its supply of required nutrients on a consistent basis, this sets you up for low level health and your body goes into survival mode. Your entire physiology gets thrown way off and now you have disequilibrium. As such, your body becomes deficient in key bio-nutrients as in minerals, trace minerals, vitamins, anti-oxidants, essential fats, enzymes and other key nutrients for creating optimum health.

Your body also becomes quite toxic as now you do not have the required bio-nutrients to remove toxins and metabolic wastes out of your system as is the natural process for keeping your body clean and healthy.

Another unhealthy factor of the food supply is that many prepared foods have toxins in them as in synthetic preservatives, binders and fillers which makes your body toxic when you ingest such food compounds. So you have 2 main factors to the food supply that make it a source of low nutrition content and can be toxic. Also, because you do not have the reserve nutrients to move toxins out of your system, your body becomes quite toxic internally over time.

Here is the secret that you need to know. In the attempt to neutralize these toxins and to protect your organs, your body will produce fat globules around these toxins. Do you get this?

What most people are unaware of is that overweight people are extremely toxic due to their daily food intake of low nutrient and toxic compounds. This is one of the main reasons why so many people are so overweight.

MSG is a synthetic compound that is being added to many foods to flavor them, however, the name is being disguised as something else and it may be a list of 100 different names. MSG is addicting and causes you to want to eat more of a food item and you will crave that food more often so you go out and buy it. Do you get it? There are also many other toxic compounds being added to foods that may contribute to weight gain as in corn syrup and cane sugar and many others.

Essentially, most of the foods on grocery store shelves contain these funny and toxic compounds. These foods cannot sustain life and are one of the causes of the great number of overweight and obese people in the world, in particular the USA. Do you see this now? Just because a food item is on a shelf does not mean it shall feed your body properly.

Also, because you are not getting the vital bio-nutrients that soil bacteria are supposed to supply produce with, your body cannot function the way it needs to. I can go on and on about this topic, however, what I have just revealed is where you need to start if you want to get results for becoming slimmer and healthier.

It starts with the decision that you are going to honor your body and not put toxic and funny food into it just as you wouldn't put something funny or toxic in the gas tank of your car. Stop putting the low quality food into your body and begin to clean your nutrition intake up. You require to intake whole-some foods that have nutrients and life to give in them. As you do, amazing things start happening to your body because now your body has nutrients to work with and not toxins.

If you are overweight, obese or simply want to get rid of cellulite, then you require to first stop eating the low nutrient and toxic foods. This is simple science. Just as your car requires the proper gas and oil for it to function right, so too does your body require the key nutrients to be healthy.

Drinking and eating foods that are devoid of key bio-nutrients puts your body in survival mode and alters your basal metabolic rate. Your basal meta-bolic rate is essentially the rate at which your body transforms calories into energy. What you must comprehend is that by eating junk food and nutrient devoid food, your metabolism gets altered in a way that actually causes your body to transform calories super slowly. **So, not only do you put your body in survival mode (storing fat – to surround the toxins to protect your organs) by eating low quality food, you also cause your metabolism to function in a slow mode which in turn causes weight gain.**

Do you see now what has been going on with you and why you haven't been able to shed weight effectively and to keep it off? It is the choices of your food intake and what those foods contain in them and the physiological effect they have on your system.

This is quite simple when you boil it down to simple science and com-mon sense. The solution is also quite simple. Actually, it is quite amazing to see people get profound results once they learn how to structure a proper nu-trition lifestyle that suits their body type.

Another main component to the obesity topic and why most people cannot reduce their weight easily is that most people are super dehydrated. You see, your body requires to be hydrated properly for 3 main reasons.

One is that water is supposed to drive nutrients to the cells of your body so there can be an exchange of energy and information from nutrients to cells. On the perimeter of each cell there are structures called receptor sites that serve to temporarily be a docking post for nutrients to attach to the cell.

There are unique receptors sites for each nutrient as in minerals, vitamins, amino acids and such. Once a nutrient has docked onto the receptor site there is an exchange of energy and information, kind of like an electrical spark if you will. This spark is vital to your cells to function properly as they now have the energy and information to be able to do the many functions that a cell is supposed to.

If you do not hydrate your body properly then your cells cannot receive this electrical spark they require to carry out their functions. Also, due to dehydration, your body will not be able to cleanse itself of toxins and metabolic wastes. Water is a cleanser and helps to drive wastes out of the body via the elimination channels.

Due to dehydration, the body becomes quite toxic as these wastes accumulate over time and as such your entire physiology gets thrown way off. As such, your hormone system and other vital systems get imbalanced and can lead to weight gain due to your metabolism being off.

Water by the way is actually a nutrient and your cells require the oxygen and the hydrogen gases for them to function properly and to have vital life force energy as to supply you with the required bioelectricity as to maintain homeostatic balance of your entire physiology. Here is what you require to know. Simply drinking more water isn't going to hydrate your body better. In fact, the main issue has to do with the water supply of modern times. Most of the water that is currently available cannot hydrate your body properly due to a number of reasons.

The first reason why most water today will not hydrate your body properly has to do with the molecular size and structuring of the individual water molecules. You see, we humans are supposed to be drinking water from nature from natural streams and rivers.

This kind of water is structured properly and has the bio-energy from Mother Earth to hydrate our bodies and supply us with energy. However, due to pollution and modern society living conditions that is no longer a possibility.

So, there is a big problem for human health because if you do not receive the proper hydration every day, your body will not be able to function properly and will not be able detox metabolic wastes and toxins out of your system. As such, you will at some point experience low level health and for most people this translates into gaining excess weight. In essence, most overweight people are carrying many pounds worth of accumulated metabolic wastes, toxins, and parasites.

So, the properly structured water is the most important aspect to health and for being slim and radiant. In fact, most people would slim down very quickly if they simply could drink this properly structured water every day as their system can now purge toxins and parasites. **Structured Water is the key my friend.** You can go https://www.rinosoriano.com/product-page/watervortexer to discover more about properly structuring your water for better hydration.

In case you don't know...water is a Sacred compound and has many qualities to it that science is just beginning to discover. You have to become conscious of how important water is to your health and for your evolution as a human being.

Your brain requires the most hydration of any organ in your body. If your brain does not receive this properly structured water each day then your Higher faculties cannot kick in. This means that your mind, body and spirit link is going to be off and your Higher gifts and talents will not be able to come through.

Your brain will simply not be able to function at the level it is supposed to and your body then will not be able to be radiantly healthy as the brain is the Master system that coordinates all bodily functions. If your brain is off then your main bodily systems will be off like your metabolism and other vital components to health.

So, properly structured water is the holistic key for transforming your health and your entire life for that matter. Water is the most important compound for all life here on planet earth. It is life giving and has many Sacred qualities that can do wonders to your health and beyond. Water has always been a main focus for many of the Indigenous cultures as they knew of how important it is to life and evolution. Our society requires to wake up and begin to clean the waters of this world if we are going to go anywhere as a species.

So, the main issue with water today is that is has been altered from its Divine structure and is also polluted. Essentially, most bottles waters are bio-energetically DEAD, meaning there is no life force in there. Life force is the holy grail of human health.

5 Holistic Facts About Water That You DO NOT Know

1) Bottled Drinking Water Is Bio-Energetically Dead = no life force, no life force means no ability to activate your body and brain for optimum functioning

2) Bottled Water Is Toxic To Your System - bottled water has plastic residues in it thus leading to a congested liver, kidneys and brain and also clogging your detox channels.

3) The obesity and health epidemics out there are a direct result of de-hydration through the ingestion of bio-energetically dead and toxic water.

4) Water that is unstructured and has plastic residues in it can not be processed by your body and thus most people are storing this toxic water outside their cells. This storing of toxic water is one of the main culprits of obesity and being overweight. This coupled with the DEAD food supply and you get a ripe condition for health epidemics.

5) Bottled water is lowering your vibration and diminishing your level of Consciousness.

It's kind of like your cell phone battery. When you have a charge and juice you can make calls, send and receive texts. What would happen if someone removed the battery from your cell phone? Would you be able to make calls, send or receive texts? No way!

Bottled water is like your cell phone without a battery, no ability to do anything because it is DEAD!

We are supposed to be drinking water from nature from running bodies of water. When water is moving along the planet, it is being kept charged and infused with life force energy.

The second you remove water from nature and it stops moving, the life force begins to dissipate. After a few days, that water is now lifeless. It can not give life any longer.

Also, anytime you run water through pipes and filter it as in reverse osmosis, distillation, alkalization and other water treatment methods, you remove the electron spin surrounding the water molecule. This removal of electrons (no energy production) from the molecules leaves water lifeless and has no ability to hydrate you nor help you create radiant health.

Water without life force is depleting to your body. Life force creates magnetic charge in water, with this magnetic charge water can now carry nutrients to your cell membranes. Also, water that has this magnetic charge is also able to attract toxins and move them out of your system for elimination.

Thus, water without life force or magnetic charge can not move nutrients to your cell membranes nor detox your body of toxins, calcification, parasites or heavy metals. Thus, you store this yucky stuff inside your body and the load gets heavier and heavier. Do you get what I am saying? Just look around at all the overweight people...they are carrying many pounds worth of heavy metals, parasites, calcification and other toxins including toxic water.

At this point in the game 90% of humans are bankrupt of vital hydration and nutrients and thus you get what you got with most people being overweight and with health epidemics that continue to rise each year. Without correcting this major problem in life, humans have no shot at being healthy nor living the life of their dreams.

Water With Life Force Creates Radiant Health & Radiant Bodies

Water with life force is the holy grail of human health. Water with life force activates your enzymes, your metabolism and your hormones and is key for activating your brain so you can access higher states of Consciousness and Higher Faculties

Pure & Structured Water is the gateway to your Highest Potentials and Highest Expansion.

The Sacred molecular structuring to water of modern society has been changed and so thus it cannot hydrate the body as it is Divinely supposed to. Anytime you run water through machines, pipes and other water systems, you change the molecular structure to it.

Many people think that drinking distilled water and reverse osmosis water is healthy...well, it is not healthy my friend. These types of water will actually over time cause you many health issues as their molecular structures are not ideal for human health. These waters may be cleaner as far as impurities go, however, the molecular structure to these waters cannot sustain life and keep your body healthy. They actually will deplete your system if you drink too much of these types of water.

Many bottled water companies are using reverse osmosis and other filtering processes. Well, if you simply do a little experiment then you will have the Truth. Simply take some litmus paper and dip into a glass of distilled water and reverse osmosis water. You will see that the water will show it is very acidic.

Water is supposed to be neutral or balanced in pH for your body. If it is too acidic, it may cause health disorders at some point. Also, you can do another experiment to validate the Truth of distilled water and reverse osmosis and if they are healthy.

Purchase some fresh cut flowers from your local store and simply place them into a small vase or glass. Then simply pour in some of your distilled water or reverse osmosis water. You will discover that in 2 days that the flowers are gone, no life left. If you could have properly structured water in the glass with the flowers you will discover that the flowers will still be alive after a week or more.

This is because the molecular structure and bioenergy will give life to the flowers even if they are cut flowers you bought at a store. This is how powerful Sacred Water is. It has the potential to make you radiantly healthy and for keeping you slim.

Let me give you some holistic science of why most water today is not able to fully hydrate your body properly. What I am explaining here is simple science my friend. You can research this if you like to validate for yourself. On a molecular level, your cells have a structure called an Aquaporin on the cell membrane.

This Aquaporin is the size of a nanometer and is designed to intake water for the cells. This means that for water to enter the cells through this Aquaporin it has to be the size of a nanometer or smaller. Now, here is where the issue is with most bottled waters and spigot water. The size of those water molecules are anywhere from ½ micron to 1 micron in size. Here is a simple formula just so you can see where the issue lies:

1000 nanometers = 1 micron

From this formula you can deduce that essentially you have 1000 nanometers that will fit into a 1 micron. **Essentially, most bottled waters and spigot waters have a molecular size that is way too BIG to enter into the aquaporin of your cells.** It is like trying to squeeze a basketball into a golf ball hole. It simply is not going to happen.

Thus, you have a big issue with health and one of the main reasons why so many people are overweight. Most people's systems are super dehydrated and toxic and thus you get what you got...a super overweight society. This is simple science my friend. I am here to shed some light on this Truth because if our society really cares for its evolution them the water supply requires resolution and I mean fast.

Fortunately, I have discovered a few inventions that can help to restructure water and make it more absorbable by your body. These devices simply help water to remember is Sacred and Divine molecular structure.

As such, when you drink water that has been structured properly, your body now can function better and begin to cleanse itself. The results speak for themselves. You can validate the results pretty quickly as your body will begin to give you signs that it is receiving more hydration.

Be aware that there are many water machines and devices out nowadays. A majority of these water machines do not structure the water to be ideal for your health. In fact some of these machines and the water they create can be unhealthy to use long term. Please contact me if you desire more scientific information about properly structured water by visiting my website at **Rino-Soriano.com**

You have to understand something and that is your body is immaculate and is very intelligent. Every single cell in your body is alive and conscious. Your cells require your help with supplying them with the appropriate compounds so they may do their functions.

The issue with modern society is that is has gotten way off path and has deviated from nature. As such, this modern society has gotten to be way too toxic and depleting. How can you expect your body to function properly if you are ingesting nutrient devoid foods and drinking water that is not hydrating???

When you go to gas up your car, you get the right octane gas in there, right? You would not put something toxic in there would you or something that is not supposed to go in there, correct? Well, each day most people are ingesting foods and drinks that are not meant to go in the human body. Again, I am simply stating facts and the Truth about health.

Give your body what it requires to function properly and the results speak for themselves. Your body can easily correct any imbalances quickly given that you supply it with the required compounds. This is so simple yet most people miss this. Society has made health so complex and confusing. You require simplifying the aspect of your health and follow natural laws and principles that validate themselves.

So, what do you choose to put into your body from now on... toxic and nutrient devoid compounds that will create low level health or life giving foods and structured water that helps your body to be healthy and radiant?

CHAPTER 2

THE HAMSTER WHEEL PARADIGMS MAKES YOU GAIN WEIGHT

Now you know the Truth of why you and so many people are over-weight and have not been able to find a solution. I will now speak about how the current weight reduction philosophies are not healthy as is being claimed. Most paradigms out there teach you too limit your fat and your calorie intake in order to reduce weight.

This may appear to be true on the surface, however, in actuality the Truth is that by limiting fat and calories you actually put your body in survival mode and will cause yourself to gain weight over the long run.

You see, your body requires a consistent supply of viable nutrition throughout the day and when you limit too much fat and calories for too long, the natural survival mechanism kicks in and slows your metabolism down in order to preserve your health. Yes you may reduce some weight by following such advice, however, what you must realize is that the weight you are losing is mainly water weight and if anything else you lose some muscle which is the last thing you want to do.

So, many people have followed the limit your calories and fat paradigms, they may have even lost some weight, however, what they did was to actually make themselves fatter proportionately speaking because now in losing water and muscle, they actually have more fat than before in fat to muscle ratios.

The order that you lose is the following: First you lose water weight, the next thing that goes is muscle and the very last thing to go is fat. If you are toxic and dehydrated then your body will let not go of the fat no matter what you do. So, if you attempt to reduce your weight the limit fat and calorie paradigm way that is taught out there, yes you may shed some weight, you get a bit smaller, however, you now have less muscle on your body which alters your basal metabolic rate to burn calories slower than before.

Do you see the funny cycle that is created here by following paradigms and so called weight reduction remedies? You must be conscious of these facts that I am presenting because you will be like a hamster on the wheel, spinning and spinning and wasting energy without True results. I think by now you get the idea and you see what I am saying.

To follow the paradigm way will eventually lead you to gain much more weight overall because once you start ingesting more calories again, due to your basal metabolic rate burning calories so slowly, you wind up gaining weight quite easily now. **You require getting off the hamster wheel and stop eating the grunge foods.**

CHAPTER 3

DEMYSTIFYING AND VAPORIZ-ING THE HEALTH MYTHS

Are you ready to discover the greatest erroneous health myths ever presented to you? Again, prepare yourself to shed these illusions as they are hindering your ability to create an optimal level of health. In fact, some of these erroneous myths have done more to keep you and other people unwell and caused you to gain weight than to benefit your health. Here we go my friend, the myths are about to be exposed and vaporized.

The Low Fat Myth

You probably may believe that it is healthy to eat a low fat diet and to limit your total fat intake each day, correct? Well, this is actually one of the greatest myths ever created. Many people have done a disservice to their health and their families by following this erroneous myth. Let me present some basic science facts for you so that you may learn to discern the Truth of this topic as it is crucial for you to know.

Regardless of what has been presented to you on this topic, the simple science fact is...**fat is the most essential nutrient your body requires for optimal health.** It is required for many processes in your body and is a precursor to hormone production.

What this means is that your body requires a consistent supply of the right kinds of fat in order for you to have the right hormone levels in your body, along with keeping your immune system strong and for skin, hair, eyes and brain health. If you reduce total fat from your diet, you are going to alter your hormone chemistry along with being deficient in essential fatty acids that are required for optimum biological processes. Thus you may experience improper health and functioning of your body. Also, fats are the greatest source of energy. Do you comprehend what this means? It means that you will actually have greater energy levels if you consume healthy fats on a consistent basis.

So, by consuming healthy levels of fat every day, you are easily increasing your energy levels. The myth that says that fat makes you fat is actually false and has been proven scientifically. **The Truth is by consuming healthy fats on a consistent basis you will actually moderate and improve your metabolism.**

This means that you will actually reduce weight or maintain a healthy weight level. Ingesting fat does not make you fat. In fact, fat breaks down into water and lipids as it goes through digestion. The water portion your body will use as hydration and the lipid portion your body will use for hormone production and other vital biological functions.

You can validate this simple Truth by embodying this information in your daily nutrition intake. Keep in mind that you require to ingest the right kinds of fats, not just any type. What has been discovered around the world is that the cultures that ingest moderate to high amounts of healthy fats are the healthiest people on the planet.

Again, this is simple science and validates itself. The fats that are harming people are the altered and hydrogenated forms. These fats are quite toxic to the system and these are the oils that are causing improper health in many people. Hydrogenated oils are super high heated and altered from their natural composition.

When you heat a compound, you alter it on a molecular level and thus create something new. In the aspect of oils, when they are heated they are changed and become toxic to your system. These oils are the ones to stay away from.

Thus, oils like margarine, Crisco, vegetable oils, canola oil, corn oil, soy oil, Wesson oil, and the whole list of altered oils are the ones to stay away from regardless of what you may think. Canola oil has been presented as a healthy oil. Well, if you do some research it has been discovered to be toxic over long term use. If you learn about where it comes from and how it is processed then the Truth is that it is not a healthy oil to consume.

Be aware that it is not healthy to cook with most oils from the fact that you alter the composition when you heat the oil.

So, my recommendation is to use steam, roasting, and grilling with a little water to cook your meals and then at the completion when your food is fully cooked after you take it off the heat, then add your oil. So, for example, if you make a soup, place all the ingredients into the pot with water and then cook it until the soup is done. Now add your oil and spices to flavor and add the healthy component of the fat. If you do require using oil to cook with, I recommend using coconut oil and grapeseed oil as these have high smoking points and can be used safely if you cook with them quickly.

Super Power Fats

The healthiest oils for health are natural, unaltered and very healthy for your body. These fats include avocado, truly raw olive oil, grapeseed oil, coconut oil, walnut oil, almond oil, and palm oil.

Now, there is another type of fat that many health paradigms are saying are very unhealthy for you and that is the class of saturated fats as in animals fats. These health paradigms claim that these fats will clog your arteries and impact your health negatively. Well, the Truth is that **saturated fats are the most essential fat required for optimum health.** They are even more essential than the healthy plant oils I mentioned earlier.

Here is the reason why: **the saturated fats are required by your body as a precursor to proper hormone production. Essentially, the saturated fats are the specific building compounds that your body requires to be able to create the chain of molecules that eventually make up your hormones.**

Hormones by the way are directly involved in almost every single biological process in your body and the main one is metabolism.

Scientifically speaking, we humans are considered animals and as such we require honoring nature's laws. For we humans to sustain our health we require to ingest animal fats. It is this simple. On a molecular level, the animal saturated fats are what the body requires to produce healthy hormone levels. Simply observe nature and the Truth is quite apparent. If you require more proof then simply research the discoveries of Weston A. Price and you will have more than enough validating information on what most humans are meant to be ingesting.

Myth #1 exposed and vaporized!

The Cardiovascular Myth

Here is another myth that has been presented as Truth, however, does not validate itself. Engaging in cardiovascular endurance activities at high levels several times per week is not conducive to optimum health. You know the activities I am talking about...aerobics, running, marathons, treadmill, and other activities and sports that result is extended elevation of heart levels. Let me clarify.

Your body is equipped with some Divine capabilities and with reserve systems that help it to function and repair. The main point here is that if you engage in high intensity cardiovascular activities on a routine basis, you are actually depleting your body and your reserves to adequately repair and regenerate.

The current health paradigm is teaching you to go out 3 to 5 days a week at 45 minutes to 1 hour to do cardio activities. It is recommended to go at 60 to 75% of maximum heart rate capability. This is ludicrous to say the least. Where this came from I have no idea but let me give you a good example of what this philosophy is saying. Essentially, it is like running your car at 75% of its maximum capability on a consistent basis.

It is like stomping on the gas pedal at a stop light to go every time. Or, another example is if you have a manual stick shift car, it is like driving your car using first and second gear only with revving the engine on a daily basis at high RPM levels. Do you think you car's engine will last long by running it in this manner? In fact, by doing this, the engine will burn out much faster.

Well, this is what people are doing to themselves by engaging in high intensity and long duration cardiovascular activities. Essentially, they are elevating their heart levels too high and potentially causing themselves harm over the long term.

In fact, if you want to shorten your life span then this is one way to do that. **So, the main point is, it is not healthy to engage in high intensity long duration activities and also unnecessary.**

Your heart doesn't require this type of stimulation to be healthy. Yes, you require being active, you just need to do it in a healthy manner. In fact, it is best to keep your heart rate at low to moderate levels when engaging in sport activities. This is why lifting weights in the right manner is the greatest activity you can do for looking and feeling your best. By lifting weights properly and for the right duration, you do so many awesome things for your health.

First, your body will produce many life regenerating hormones that will keep you young looking and feeling young. Second, you will put on muscle mass which in turn will help to keep your weight healthy by moderating your metabolism and you get the benefit of looking awesome.

How amazing that a simple activity like lifting weights can do so many awesome things for your health. This is the #1 activity to engage in if you want to add many years to your life.

There are also other processes going on with working out with weights as in strengthening your ligaments and tendons and also mental and emotional components that most people have no clue that comes from lifting weights.

Again, you require to lift weights in the right manner otherwise, you are wasting time, money and energy. I can show anyone how to do it in the right manner. It is actually so simple yet most people are unaware.

What they teach at the gym, well, this is not very effective for most people because it is over working your muscles and then the nutrition habits of most people does not support maximum gains in health and building muscle. I will now give you a simple example that shall help you to see the Truth of how high endurance long duration activities are not healthy.

If you simply observe the difference between a marathon runner and a sprinter the Truth becomes quite apparent. Whom do you think is healthier and has a better functioning body? The Truth is that the sprinter is way healthier than the marathon runner. In fact, not even close. The marathon runner is depleted and week compared to the sprinter. The marathon runner's activity and lifestyle don't allow for the body to recuperate or regenerate so thus they are in a catabolic (weak, degenerating) state.

In essence, their training and their activity is too depleting on the body and is never allowed to recuperate properly, thus simply looking at them will tell the tale and the Truth of the matter. The sprinter on the other hand is in anabolic phase and as is quite evident by simply observing their body, they are quite healthy looking and feeling.

These athletes have high power, strength and musculature. Their body is in anabolic phase meaning they are regenerating and building muscle on a routine basis. **Their activity is short duration and so is their training. This is the key and one of the main secrets for engaging in fitness activities.**

You see, the body absolutely requires to be worked out, however, you require to do it in the right manner otherwise it has the opposite effect. Your muscles and body have only so many available nutrients, hydration and ATP energy to perform in activities. The intention is to engage in activities where you are using readily available bio-nutrients that your body has to give.

You want to avoid engaging in either long duration sports or activities or high intensity activities that cause you to dip into your reserve supply of energy and nutrients. This is why most athletes have short careers because they consistently place their body into tapping into reserves and they never allow their body to recuperate adequately.

The main key is to engage in activities that are short duration or start stop sports. Sports like tennis, volleyball, lifting weights, pilates, hiking, power walking and other similar short duration or start stop activities are ideal for optimal health. These activities do not stimulate your heart and do not cause your body to dip into reserves as much as other sports. The other main key is to fully allow the body to recuperate after engaging in your activity.

The secret is you can actually get in better shape by let's say working out with weights for only 25 to 30 minutes than if you spend 1 hour or more as most people do. In fact, the results are quite amazing when you see someone who does the proper weight training program as I teach, and the results they get with actually doing less.

So, my main point to you is…yes engage in activities and do them on a consistent basis, however, reduce the sports that will deplete you. Also, re-member to allow full recovery after your sports.. Most people do not know how to do this properly. This is important if you want to regenerate and extend your life span.

It is important to structure your nutrition intake as to replenish and regenerate your body properly along with using the right supplements for muscle recovery. As shall be presented throughout this book, you will be given the keys on how to do this more efficiently as to maximize results. **Myth #2 Vaporized!**

The Cholesterol Myth

In recent years the talk about cholesterol and how you need to limit total levels every day for better health. Really? No thanks...just another funny myth my friend! Here is another erroneous theory that has no scientific basis whatsoever. Once again, people have done themselves a great disservice by following such crap. Pay attention because I keep things very simple.

Cholesterol is a required compound for optimum health. You need to ingest it in sufficient levels to maintain proper functioning of your body. It has numerous functions to keeping you young looking, vital and feeling healthy. The simple fact is, if you ingest the right kinds of fats then you will receive the healthy cholesterol type that benefits your health and longevity. If you do not ingest the right kind of cholesterol then you are doing yourself a disservice.

The harmful cholesterol only comes from hydrogenated oils and fats that are chemically altered from their natural state. So, the key is to eat the right kinds of oils and fats and do it on a consistent basis. You won't have to ever worry about getting high cholesterol levels because your body will moderate it just fine because you are ingesting the right fats. If you ingest the wrong kinds of fats then that is when you will get high cholesterol levels.

So do yourself a favor, keep it simple and eat the right kinds of fats, very easy and simple to follow. Leave the rest, don't buy the hype of erroneous health paradigms out there. There is no need to worry about high cholesterol levels if you eat a balanced and natural diet for your body type. **Another erroneous myth exposed and vaporized!**

The Eat Lean Meats Myth

In recent years there has been a shift of people starting to eat leaner cuts of meat such as chicken breast, lean red meat portions and other meats of leaner type. It is proposed that eating leaner meats is healthier than eating fattier portions of meat as in chicken wings and chicken legs and rib eye steaks and ground beef.

Well my friend, yep you guessed it, just another erroneous myth being proposed as healthy. Let me simply provide basic holistic facts and common sense because that is all you require to see the Truth.

Eating lean cuts of meats actually promotes low levels of health and causes your body to become depleted of nutrients and creates an acidic environment internally. Lean meat is pure protein and requires extra enzymes and other bio-nutrients to break down the protein so that your body may make use of it to supply itself for nutrition.

Excessive consumption of lean meats causes all sorts of health disorders and places strain on the liver and colon. By the way, eating fatty portions of meat DOES NOT clog arteries as is being proposed. The clogged arteries come from other factors such as the consumption of unhealthy hydrogenated fats, excessive sugar intake which leads to yeast and parasite formation and other metabolic wastes in the body that accumulate in the heart ventricles.

You may actually get artery clogging by ingesting excessive amounts of lean meats since the body becomes acidic and then your body will have to take calcium from your system. Calcium is the main buffer mineral used by the body to neutralize acids and other harmful waste products. After some time of this process of using calcium to buffer acids there are bio-wastes that will accumulate in your system and usually the heart area is where it coagulates and becomes like stones and other hard deposits. So in essence you are doing yourself a disservice by consuming lean portions of meats.

The Truth is that eating the fattier portions of meats as in chicken wings and legs and the inners of the chicken, rib eye steaks, ground beef (the fattier the better) and other fatty meats is absolutely healthy and promote good health. Research Weston A. Price Foundation and you will have your validations and more.

The main thing is to moderate your portions. A portion the size of your hand is a great guide to follow when eating meats. Also be sure to balance your meal with enough fresh veggies. In fact, **my recommendation is to always have half of your plate be fresh steamed veggies.**

The main issue of today and why people are experiencing health disorders is that they have their portions and their meat options way off. They are eating big portions of lean meats, a large serving of starch food and a super small portion of vegetable. This ratio of nutrition causes acidity in the body which leads to numerous health disorders and places undue stress on your organs. The key is to alter the ratios and the meats options and then you are on the right track.

A healthy meal consists of a half plate of fresh steamed veggies or raw, a complex starch food as in quinoa, brown rice or wild rice, sweet potato or gluten free or sprouted bread and then a small portion of fatty meat as in chicken legs or rib eye steak. This meal is balanced and has the proper ratio of fats to starches to protein.

Also, another fact to become aware of is that eating fattier portions of meats is actually easier on your body. Fatty meat is easier to digest and requires less enzymes and bio-nutrients to break down. And...the secret that your body knows which is healthier...the fatty meat. This is so simple but again you have been programmed to go against what nature has intended. So, do yourself a simple experiment...or even just think about it in a common sense way...if you have 2 options before you, one is a plate of lean chicken breast and the other plate has 3 chicken legs...which does your body feel a pull toward? Which do you really want to eat? Which tastes better and feels better when you eat it? Pretty simple!

Another funny myth exposed and vaporized. Ah...Ba Bye!

CHAPTER 4

THE COMPOUNDS THAT MAKE YOU GAIN WEIGHT

The following so called foods are ones that will put weight on your body easily as they cause your body to be toxic and have a negative physiological effect on your metabolism.

Corn Syrup – any time you ingest anything with corn syrup, the physiological effect on your body is that it is toxic to your system and will convert this right to fat because of the molecular structure to the sugars.

Your body will gain more weight by drinking soda or any other sweetened drink than food. Beer also causes rapid weight gain since it gets converted to sugar in your body and then alters your metabolism. Beer also promotes the growth of parasites.

You will also gain weight easily every time you ingest anything with processed sugar. Processed sugar is not meant to go in the body. It is actually quite toxic to your system. The molecular structure and composition to the sugar is not healthy and it actually degenerates the body.

It makes your body acidic and stimulates your nervous system. It gives you a false energy by stimulating your brain and nervous system. So, in actuality, consuming any processed forms of sugar depletes you of energy and nutrients because of the physiological effect on the body.

Again, sugar is toxic to your system and thus your body attempts to neutralize the toxic effects. Sugar also promotes the growth of parasites and yeast (fungi). Many people of today have lots of parasites and fungi which in turn put out their own toxins into your system which in turn may cause more weight gain. As I have already revealed, your body produces fat globules around toxins to neutralize them from doing your organs harm.

Parasites can also cause your brain chemistry to be altered and they may even cause you to crave specific sweet foods. Parasites feed off of processed sugars of any form. They contribute to making your system toxic and may cause you weight gain or at least make losing weight a challenge.

White flour products also contribute to weight gain. These foods contain no nutrients other than starches which in turn break down into sugars in your body when you ingest them. Did you get that? By eating white flour products, the physiological effect on your body is that your system will convert it to sugar which then gets converted to fat in your body.

Many white flour products also contain sugar as an ingredient which makes that food product a double whammy because you have in actuality a product of high dose sugar once you ingest it. Both will get converted to fat in your body.

These foods also promote parasite growth since the flour gets converted to sugar once in your body. Again, this is a cycle that is self-feeding as long as you keep ingesting high sugar, white flour, and low quality foods and drinks. You require getting off the cycle completely if you want any resolution whatsoever.

If you can remove just 2 compounds from your diet, you will immediately feel the difference. Removing white flour products and any and all products that contain any form of processed sugars shall do wonders to your health and shall make losing weight much simpler.

Due to sugar being so toxic and stimulating to your system, it can cause your hormones to be thrown off key. Hormones govern your metabolism and thus you alter your metabolism by ingesting too much sugar or starchy food products.

Sweetened drinks are the worst compound to ingest as they profoundly alter your inner ph and physiology. This in turn can alter your hormones and eventually your metabolism. The drinks with corn syrup and other sweeteners in society that are so popular will cause you more weight gain and faster than anything else.

My recommendation is stay away from all sweetened drinks, even natural and organic juices and teas. These drinks are way too concentrated and can really mess up your hormones and physiology. It is not worth it.

Sodas are by far the worst sweetened drink as they have many negative factors as in they are loaded with sugar, they have phosphorous which is very acidic to your body and the carbonation is also a very acidic compound to your body. This makes this kind of drink a super unhealthy compound that has many negative implications to your health and well-being.

Sugar Impacts Your Evolution Negatively

Ingesting sugar can also stifle your Higher Faculties of Intuition and other Spiritual Abilities. Its impact on the brain is very unhealthy and causes the brain chemistry to be thrown way off.

Your brain is functioning at a multi-dimensional level and processing Higher Dimensional information along with governing your entire body physiology. Ingesting sugar essentially does not allow your brain to connect to your Higher Faculties which you require to evolve yourself.

To evolve you require to be tapped into your Higher Faculties of Intuition and other Higher Faculties. With sugar in your diet, you are doing a great disservice to your body and also to your evolution. Here is the main reason: **Your cells and DNA are supposed to be vibrating at faster than the speed of light.** Yes this is a fact! If you truly comprehend just how complex your body is and how many biological processes are occurring in each second then you will see that having your cells vibrating at the speed of light or lower is too slow for your body to function optimally.

You see, your cells require information in a steady stream of pulsing energies or what some call Chi. In essence, your entire physiology is running via energy in the form of information coming from your brain as a direct link from Universal Consciousness or Source.

The speed at which this happens is way beyond the speed of light, in fact probably a multiple thereof. It has to be at this super-fast speed in order for your entire body cellular system to receive all of the vast quantity of information coming in.

Here is a secret for you: When the cells and DNA of the body vibrate slower than the speed of light, this is when health disorders begin to set in.

The relay of vital information your cells require to function optimally is simply too slow for your major systems to keep everything flowing as is Divinely intended.

Picture your wireless internet connection and when things are ideal you have super-fast loading and processing and everything is good. However, what happens if your internet connection begins to get bogged down and your computer starts to slow up and you cannot even load websites or check email. You have had this happen before and it makes your internet experience not fun.

Well, this is what happens when your body, cells and DNA are vibrating below the speed of light. Your cells simply cannot function as they are supposed to as the relay of vital energy and information that each cells requires is way too slow for optimum functioning. Do you see this? I pray you do because maybe, just maybe, you will begin to change your perspective on your health and your body?

Ingesting sugar literally slows the vibration of your cells and DNA below the speed of light and thus sets you up for low level health.

By the way, your DNA is so much more than some base nucleotides as modern science says. Your DNA is multi-dimensional and is also processing information from Source. There are components to DNA that cannot been seen by human eyes or microscopes, however, if you truly comprehend what DNA really is and what it really is doing you would marvel. Your DNA is actually like a multi-dimensional super computer and is constantly changing.

How does it change you may ask? It changes as you change. It changes with every thought you have, with every mood you have, it changes with what is going on in your environment as in the space you live and where you work. Do you comprehend what this means?

My friend, your DNA is constantly changing based on the frequencies and energies you are supplying it with via your thoughts, emotions, nutrition, your home environment, your work place, your friends, the music you listen to, the tv programs you watch, the clothes you wear and even the people you live with.

Maybe this is the motivation you require to do a complete holistic lifestyle makeover? Until you understand life on this profound level as I am presenting to you then you will probably not make the changes in your life to experience shifts that will catapult your evolution.

This is why what I teach about holistic living is so profound, because it helps you to shift at the most profound levels and ensures you only input healthy frequencies and energies in, on and around your body as to help you to experience Higher levels of health and wellness. My friend, it is the only way for you to even begin to tap into your Higher Potentials.

In essence, your body and your level of health is a direct link to your evolution as a human being and for being able to tap into your Higher Potentials.

The healthier you are, the more you can tap into Higher Faculties and Higher Gifts and Talents as they will be able to come through since your cells and DNA are vibrating at faster than speed of light. Thus, Higher Dimensional information will be able to be processed by your brain and thus allow you to perform and do things that most people simply cannot do.

You will surprised to see just how much better you feel by simply removing all forms of processed sugar from your diet. In fact, within a few days you will feel a new sense of relief and calm and well-being.

There are many other food items that will have similar physiological effects on your body as sugar does. Most people are simply unaware that everything you ingest breaks down into smaller components. Many food items that people ingest actually will break down into sugar-like compounds.

Food items such as white flour products, white rice, cereal, potato chips, pretzels, corn chips, crackers and other dry brittle food items will get converted into sugar once in your body. As such, the physiological effect is that these food items can actually cause you to gain weight due to the effect on your metabolism and inefficient functioning of your entire biological system.

These processed food items are not nutrition for your body and will only serve to lower your level of health. My recommendation is to stay away from these food items as there are far healthier alternatives.

I have written a recipe called **Fun Food Fantastic** that has some of the most knock your socks off meal creations. I have in the recipe book super delicious and healthy recipes that will satisfy your taste buds and be healthy for your body. You can go here to my Amazon Book Page www.amazon.com/-/e/B009I7K4MA or my website to download it.

CHAPTER 5

MENTAL, EMOTIONAL AND SPIRITUAL FACTORS TO WEIGHT GAIN

I am here to be honest with you and so at this time I want to clarify an important topic. I think you require to be made aware of this since it can mean a huge difference in the results you experience on your journey to a healthier and slimmer you. This I believe is the missing component to experiencing the Highest results in your total life. It is also the secret key for transforming the real cause to your weight gain.

You see, you are a multi-dimensional being. You have a physical complex and also a mental, emotional and spiritual complex that makes you uniquely you. To concentrate strictly on the physical aspect of your being will only give you limited results. The reason is because your mental, emotional and spiritual aspects to your being have a much bigger impact on your health than do physical factors alone. Do you get this? How you respond to life emotionally and mentally will have more pull on your health than just your physical self.

What most people miss is that these unseen aspects to your being require love, nurturing and nourishment as well. Most people have mental and emotional issues that they are carrying.

These feelings deep inside require to be honored and expressed otherwise they impact your health in negative ways and can be the True cause for your weight gain. You see, if you have inner unresolved issues, these feelings will cause you to unconsciously behave in ways that are not healthy such as eating foods that are comforting which are mainly full of sugar, salt and preservatives.

They are called comfort foods because they temporarily give you some good feelings because they impact your brain, however, the good feelings only last a short time. As such, you require to continue eating these unhealthy foods to get the great brain feeling.

This unconscious behavior and the unresolved inner feelings are the True cause of weight gain for most people. This may apply to you or not, however, everything in life is symbolic and you require sitting with yourself and be honest. How do you really feel deep inside? How do you feel about yourself, really? How do you view life? Do you view it as a beautiful experience or do you view it otherwise.

Your inner belief system is very powerful and can cause you to say and do things that you wouldn't if you were a bit more conscious of your inner emotional, mental and spiritual self. So, sit with yourself and begin to see what unresolved issues you may have.

You see, most people want to numb or cover over these inner feelings so they may tend to do that with food. So, they go for the food that is usually the real salty, sugary and yummy stuff since it gives them a temporary feeling of goodness. This behavior works unconsciously and until you become conscious of what you are doing and why, you will continue to follow the same behavior.

Just as a rock thrown into a pond causes a ripple of the water to go out and affect the entire pond, so too do your inner mental, emotional and spiritual aspects of your being ripple out to affect your full being of mind, body and spirit. Do you see this?

So, if you want to experience great results in your healthy lifestyle then you require looking inside yourself and begin to detox the outdated and unresolved feelings from your life. Most of these unresolved issues come from childhood so I recommend having a coach walk you through a process to keep things structured and on path.

Look, I want you to be happy and be radiantly healthy and in order for you to do that, you require to look at all aspects of you being. This is why I am presenting this topic to you since most people miss this and experience limited results. I want you to be the healthiest possible because you benefit everyone on the planet when you are.

When you are radiantly healthy, you walk with a new sense of energy, of purpose and you want to go out in life and rock it by doing amazing things. You also serve as an example for others to begin their healing. Please for your sake and the whole of humanity, begin your path to healing. It gets easier as you clean your life up and eat cleaner. You simply require the proper path to follow.

Once you are on a structured path that gets results then with each step, you become more and more confident and more inspired to keep going.

I think you see the connection of how inner unresolved feelings can be the cause of your desire to want to eat the unhealthy foods. If you research the topic of metaphysics or mind science, you shall discover that they show that unresolved life issues result in unconscious behaviors and also health conditions. These behaviors and health conditions come up to make you conscious that something is going on within you and it requires your love and attention.

So, in the aspect of health and weight gain, fat is actually a buffer if you will. It serves to protect the organs and to provide you energy in case you require it for times you may not eat for a time period. These are both for protection, to help keep you healthy and safe.

Well, in the metaphysical viewpoint, if you are overweight then this symbolizes that you are protecting yourself from something as to provide a buffer from getting hurt. So subconsciously you may have created a belief somewhere in your life, usually in childhood that says you require protecting yourself. Your subconscious mind wants to protect you and so thus it does everything it can to do that.

On a subconscious level, if you carry a belief that you require to protect yourself then your mind will symbolically do that. Thus, you unconsciously begin eating unhealthy foods that contribute to weight gain to provide you the safety buffer (fat). If you research data on the subconscious mind you shall discover many examples of how the subconscious mind symbolically creates situations to protect you.

The time has come for you to take a stand and begin your path to wellness, to a healthier and slimmer you. Are you ready? Great! I am now going to lay out the foundation of what you must do to experience the resolution and the results you have been wanting. These are actually quite simplistic, however, because you have been programmed to believe otherwise, it may take a bit of time for you to embody and believe the following knowledge. Keep in mind that you have been following habits for some time now, so it shall require consistent conscious awareness (consciousity) and the intention to keep progressing.

As you continue to be consistent with your intentions while also being conscious of the path you are following, this creates a powerful synergy that compounds and gets results. The results you experience are determined by you and how far do you want go and how healthy and radiant do you want to be?

Getting the results you desire are absolutely attainable, however, the question is...are you willing to walk the path to getting there? That is something only you can say.

To begin your path to a healthier and slimmer you, I recommend to begin sitting with yourself and write down any and all feelings of unresolved life issues. It usually is one or more people that you have issues with. In some way they did or said something that impacted you. The feelings about those people require to be addressed because they are the contributing factor to your being overweight.

So, write down what you think those feelings are, is it sad, is it angry, is it confused. Write them down. Next, begin to talk to these feelings as if they are a person. Ask them what they want and what can you do to help them to express themselves. Write down what comes. Sometimes simply honoring the feelings and just allowing them to express themselves resolves them and you begin to feeling better.

Give it a try and see. The main point here is that the unresolved inner feelings require being expressed and transformed because they are the root. If you want lasting results and fantastic health levels then this process is essential. Do this process for a few weeks on a daily basis and see what shifts may occur for you. You can always say that you love them (the feelings) and honor them.

Give your feelings acknowledgment and learn to listen to what they are teaching you. Sometimes they will reveal some real powerful life wisdom that can help you in many areas of life. Become a student of your inner self because there is some powerful knowledge and wisdom in there. You will be surprised at what you learn when you are sincere and honest with doing this work.

Wisdom of The Universe

Here is what I discovered on my journey of life. Of all things I teach this is by far the most important key to life you will ever hear so do please take a few moments to allow the profundity of this revelation to inspire you to Greater Heights.

When You Are Not In Alignment With Who Your Truly Are, That Is When Your Life Simply Does Not Flow, Does Not Feel Good and You Experience Challenges.

Let me clarify for you. You see, you are a Divine Being and the Creator only creates perfect things whether this amazing Universe or a person like you. Life is about flow, expansion and evolution. However, humanity has forgotten this Sacred Truth of who they Truly are.

In doing so they have created stories of who they think they are and what they think life is supposed to be like. Instead of allowing life and the Universe to be the teachers, humanity has created man-made beliefs systems and paradigms that are not based on Truth or Substance.

As such, what you see in society is a direct reflection of what happens when humans do not honor or follow Sacred Truth or Universal Life Principles. In following illusionary philosophies, humans have created limiting stories about who they think they are and this has caused most of humanity to believe a lie about themselves.

In the aspect of your being overweight, you have created an illusionary story of who you think you are. **The larger you are in weight, the further you have deviated from your True Being.**

The more you have created such limiting beliefs about yourself and thus you see and feel this deviation in the form of your body and emotions. These are a BIG sign that you are not being who you Truly are. You have created illusionary stories based on the feedback from others as in your family members, your peers and other people whom you have interacted with in your life.

Usually in childhood, due to disharmony in the family and the lack of meeting of childhood needs, you began to create illusionary beliefs about yourself and life. As such, you are now living those belief systems of what you think life is and who you think you are.

If you are only a bit overweight then this may not apply, however, one thing is clear and that is most obese people have inner subconscious feelings about their childhood and a story that is so far from the Truth. **The Truth being that you are a Sacred Being of Love and Light and The Creator created you to be perfect.**

If you are not embodying that belief and frequency then life is going to wallop you over and over again until you wake up and drop the story and literally shed the illusions. In doing so, you will begin to shed the weight that has for so long been your life burden.

When You Are In Alignment With Who You Truly Are, The Universe Supports You Unconditionally and Floods Your Life With Beautiful Experiences.

Live True to who you are and life blesses you over and over again. When you believe your story over Sacred Truth of the Creator you will continue to get walloped. You are living a life that others may have imposed on you, you are perhaps living a life that you really do not want or a life you think you want.

However, **when you honor your True Being and live the life you truly desire, this is when your life flows and the Universe blesses you time and time again.** The Universe wants greatly for you to remember who you truly are and live that truth every day. The Universe wants you to be blissed out of your mind.

Until you surrender your story and your belief systems, then the Universe will continue to serve you what you are blipping out as the Universe is your mirror and is only reflecting back to you what you are feeling deep inside about yourself and life.

Perhaps now that you are aware of this you can begin writing a new story, a new expression of who you Truly are and allow the Universe to reveal to you by reflection your True Beauty and True Essence?

My friend, please for your sake and that of the entire planet, begin to shed your story and your illusionary belief systems as they are the stiflers that have for so long sabotaged your life and made you obese. You no longer require the story, you no longer require the fat to protect you from anyone or anything. You no longer have to put yourself through this challenge as now you are reminded of Sacred Truth and that is…**You Are Divine, You Are Sacred, You Are An Angel Star!!!**

Begin embodying this Sacred Truth and your life will now express new experiences and new feelings and new potentials.

You have played your role in your story for so long that you have simply forgotten your Inner Truth. You have fallen asleep and were simply dreaming an illusion, it is not real. Time to wake up sweet Angel Star! Clean yourself off from the muck of your story and walk out into the world with the Truth that you are Divine and Sacred. As you do, the Universe will reflect back to you your new expression. It is Law!!!

Align With Your True Self & Live Your Truth and Life Will Magically Reveal To You The Beauty of The Universe.

On this grand awakening day, I now grant you permission to drop your story, I grant you permission to shed all the illusions you have created about yourself, I grant you permission to shed the weight as you no longer require protection, I grant you permission to rise and step into your Great Beingness of who you Truly are, I grant you permission to shine your light like the sun for all to see and feel.

You are hereby granted Universal Permission to go out in life and express who you Truly are. **Happy Shining Sweet Angel Star!!!!!!!!!!!!!!!!!!!!!!!!!!!**

CHAPTER 6

STRUCTURING A SOUND HOLISTIC NUTRITION LIFESTYLE

The next step on your path to a healthier and slimmer you is to begin eliminating the foods and drinks that are contributing to your weight issues. This is a process that requires to be done properly because to eliminate only a few items is not going to get you results as you have already proven to yourself.

In essence, you require a whole nutrition and lifestyle makeover.

In order for you to get lasting results then you require to follow nutrition intake and a lifestyle that supports those results. So, the main foods and drinks to eliminate are: all white refined food products, all food products containing processed sugar in any form including corn syrup, cane juice, powdered sugar, and fructose.

White pasta and white rice are foods to eliminate as well as these get converted to sugar in your body. Also eliminate all sweetened drinks -even fruit juices, alcohol such as beer, wine and liquor as these get converted to sugar in your body which then get converted to fat.

Drink natural herbal teas or coconut water kefir instead. You can also squeeze some fresh lemon juice in your water bottle and sip this throughout the day.

Also eliminate all foods that contain any of the refined oils such as canola, corn, vegetable, margarine, soybean, Crisco, and any other hydrogenated oil as an ingredient. These oils make your body toxic and can also contribute to weight gain.

The next step is incorporating the foods that will supply you with nutrients and will help with vaporizing the fat off your body. The following food groups are essential in your life makeover: wholesome foods such as **fresh & frozen vegetables and fresh fruits, high quality oils as in coconut oil, grapeseed oil, Organic pure olive oil, avocado, sprouted nuts, almond butter, cashew butter, and raw tahini, gluten free breads, sprouted whole grain breads, whole grain gluten-free flours, pasture butter, select portions of fatty meats as in free-range chicken legs and wings, free range rib eye steaks and ground beef, lamb, and Alaskan salmon.**

The fatty portions of meat are actually the healthiest to eat, they are easier to digest and contain healthy fats that you require for a healthy body. These fats will also help you to reduce weight effectively in conjunction with the other daily habits you embody.

You require learning how to structure your nutrition intake properly as to get maximum results. You also require eating at proper times for your body type and lifestyle. My recommendation is to eat at least 3 holistically structured meals per day with at least one piece of fruit for the day. Make sure to eat mild sweet fruits only as in apples, pears, blueberries, raspberries, kiwi, strawberries.

By balancing your meals you ensure supplying your body with adequate nutrients and protein to help with your weight goals. Each meal requires to be structured as to provide a balance of fats, proteins and carbohydrates.

For example, a holistically structured meal is the following: half of your plate ought to be a vegetable of some kind for every meal, the other half of your plate then gets a half of protein and the other half is a complex carbohydrate.

This is a balanced meal and is the healthiest way of eating since vegetables contain minerals and fiber for regularity, the protein food supplies you with amino acids for rebuilding and the complex carbohydrates supply you energy.

You require including a healthy fat in this meal so thus you can add grapeseed oil, coconut oil, olive oil or butter to your steamed veggies or brown rice. The oil or butter will also supply your body with energy and shall help to give you lasting energy and strength throughout the day.

A Holistically Structured Meal:

Breakfast

- Half a plate of steamed broccoli with pink salt and onion powder

- Half of a half plate (3 eggs) of omelet with onions and pepper

- Half of a half plate (1 to 2 slices) of sprouted whole grain bread with coconut oil

This meal is balanced and contains awesome nutrients and proteins for a healthy and radiant body. The key is to make half your plate of vegetables on all main meals. This shall do wonders in helping you to lose weight and reset your metabolism for optimum functioning.

Lunch

- Half a plate of steamed green beans with pink Himalayan salt and spices

- Half of a half plate of sprouted grain bread or gluten free brown rice bread (2 slices) with avocado, cheese, tomato, with veganaise (I recommend the Follow Your Heart Brand – the lime green cap one since this one contains no soy or funny oils)

This meal is once again holistically balanced and contains vital nutrients and proteins to provide you energy and for rebuilding your body. You shall see that as you continue to eat in this fashion, your metabolism will begin to reset itself and you will actually start losing weight naturally even though you are eating more calories and more food during the day. So much for the funny paradigm that says to limit your calories and fat. Vaporize that scam right now because that has caused you and millions of people to become fatter and unhealthy. Let go of that right now and let the Truth show you the validation of what is right.

Dinner

- Half of a plate of steamed or grilled zucchini with a dash of Himalayan salt

- Half of a half plate of wild rice with sea salt and grapeseed oil

- Half of a half plate of Free-Range Chicken legs (3 legs pieces)

This meal here is balanced and will help you to improve your metabolism for a healthier and slimmer you. I have just given you a sample of one day worth of meals that is ideal for you and millions of people who are looking for a fun, delicious and healthy way to intake nutrition. I believe that nutrition ought to be fun, delicious and healthy for everyone. The intention is to create a nutrition lifestyle that embodies this strategy of eating holistically.

I can do this for anyone and create super fun, yummy and healthy meal options. It is quite easy once you see how this way of eating is the way most people ought to eat since it is balanced and supplies your body with vital nutrition.

Be aware that your health is actually fluid and changes throughout the year and throughout your life. So, you may require adjusting your nutrition intake as you sense these changes. Maybe one week your body wants more fresh fruits and streamed veggies and less meat or protein. Another week your body may require more protein since you are into working out. Learn to listen to your body as it shall guide you to what you require for nutrition intake.

CHAPTER 7

TIME FOR A COMPLETE BODY DETOX

As you begin to intake better nutrition and readjust your basal metabolic rate, now is the time to begin to purge, cleanse and detox your body of all the toxicities that it has accumulated over the years. Pay attention because there are many detox products and kits out there.

Most of these products are not worth investing in. The ones that are good simply don't provide enough detox compounds to get the job done the way you want it. In essence, to cleanse your body properly it is going to take some time over a few months at the very least. The kits at stores are for 3 to 5 to 7 days at most.

Also, you require cleansing in the proper order using the proper compounds that do what they are supposed to. Do NOT go at this detox process on your own because you will spend lots of money and get minimal results. Also, once you begin to move toxins out of your body you require supporting your body adequately because detoxing takes some energy and lots of key nutrients.

As you begin to move out heavy metals and parasites, you require supporting nutrients that will help to move this stuff out along with drinking **structured water** intake and the right moving substances. Without this knowledge you are going to waste time, money and energy and you may feel a bit off for a while.

So, do contact me if you are ready to make the decision to change your life. Be aware that most nutrition consultants and personal trainers and other health consultants are not aware of what I am revealing about weight gain and how to properly get it off.

These people mean well, however they have been taught to view things in particular ways and to recommend specific regimens that are a one size fits all. This approach will not get you results since it is based on the funny paradigm of limiting calories and fat and as I have already revealed, this way is counterproductive.

So, cleansing your body is a must if you want to truly get maximum results in losing weight and becoming slimmer and fit. As you eliminate these toxins, parasites and heavy metals from your body, you will begin to feel lighter, more energy, your consciousness levels will increase, you will be more in tune with your body and you will begin to see with your own eyes that your weight starts coming off easier.

This is due to your body now being able to let go of the fat because it doesn't need protection from those toxins. You see this right? In fact, detoxing your body is the greatest process you can do for your health and well-being. It is something you just have to experience and the results shall speak for themselves.

If you cleanse properly then the results will be profound. However, you require walking the path every day and keep on track. As you see and feel the results you will want to keep walking because it becomes self-inspiring and self-motivating. **Happy Cleansing!**

CHAPTER 8

THE 5 KEYS TO BECOMING SLIM-MER AND HEALTHIER

#1 - Begin sitting with yourself and discover what inner feelings and life issues require resolution. Go about expressing and transforming those inner feelings to a Higher expression of love and forgiveness. Contact me and I shall give you the appropriate resources for going through this process efficiently.

#2 - Begin to remove from your diet and daily nutrition intake all the toxic and nutrient devoid foods that are contributing to your weight gain and low level health.

#3 - Begin ingesting the quality foods that are life supporting and shall help you to be healthier and reset your metabolism.

#4 – Detox/Cleanse your body properly and support as you go through this process.

#5 - Engage in some form of fitness activity in the form of lifting weights, hiking, yoga, pilates, power walking or simply gardening.

This process I have just outlined is actually super simple, however, it may take you some time to adjust to because you have been following habits for some time. The intention is to just start walking and no matter what comes up, keep walking the path because it gets easier and easier as you do so. This is why it is essential for you to have the proper guidance and support while you go through this process. The guidance and support shall help you to keep on path and to remain inspired to keep walking. **Happy Walking!**

The Mysterious Demystified

A simple formula for you to follow to ensure you remain on track for optimum health is as follows: There are only 3 factors that are the cause for health disorders and low level health.

Toxins – these include heavy metals, viruses, parasites

Nutrient Deficiencies – these include water, vitamins, minerals, trace elements, essential fatty acids, amino acids, anti-oxidants, sunlight

Emotional, mental and spiritual deficiencies – resolving these can dramatically improve your health and well-being.

The time has come where each human being take responsibility for their whole lives. **Your health is the greatest asset you have.** With optimal health you can then go out and experience this life with a Higher consciousness and a great feeling. You will also be inspired to do great things as your feeling of health and wellness shall cause your Higher faculties to kick in and serve as fuel for your spiritual evolution.

It is quite amazing to see when someone is radiantly health. You can see it in their eyes and feel it in their vibration. They simply are fun to be around and get stuff done. They are creative and always looking to help people, animals and planet. These are quite extraordinary people and when you meet one of them you absolutely know as they have something remarkable about them.

Well, you can be one of these people my friend. You have the potential. **The question is...are you willing to do what it takes to be one?**

CHAPTER 9

JOIN THE HOLISTIC SLIMMING REVOLUTION

I am now going to offer you a mission of monumental proportions. Please listen carefully. My mission is to empower as many people as possible to feel and look their best. The more people that feel and look awesome the better for the entire planet.

You see, radiantly healthy people are magnetic, they have a unique style to them. They get stuff accomplished in powerful ways. They have a happy glow about them and carry themselves confidently. You have met people like this, right? Of course you have.

Well, my friend, you have this possibility yourself. You see, as you begin to feel and look better, you will also start having these qualities because it is the way all humans are supposed to be like. Everyone is supposed to feel healthy, feel radiant and happy. However, this modern society has gotten a bit toxic to say the least. In following the modern ways people have forgotten simple Truth.

The greatest health secret is that nature has all the keys for feeling and looking your best. Humanity has allowed itself to fall into illusions and scams and deceptions. In doing so, people have forgotten how to take care of their own health. This is so simple yet most people do things every day that are counter health.

I can go on and on about this subject, however, my intention is to help you because I care about humanity and I shall not sit by and watch people go through tribulations because I have the knowledge to help millions of people quite effectively.

My challenge to you is this...make the decision right now to wake up from your sleep and begin walking the path to a healthier and happier you. The path is here, however, you require walking it day after day. Only you can make this choice. You see, by you being absolutely healthy, you then can go out and be who you are meant to be.

You can experience life on a whole new level, in fact quantum leaps Higher than most. As you go out and radiate your new level of health, you will inspire people in your life to want the same. You can then help those people to change their life and walk it because you will have the knowledge and wisdom to do that.

This creates a ripple effect of positive energy and impacts many peoples' lives. This is how we are going to change this beautiful planet we call home. It takes you to make the decision to change your life and with that decision you have the potential to impact thousands of people. This is where everything is going anyway. More and more people are awakening and beginning to make healthier choices and living healthier lifestyles. Join the revolution today because the sooner you do the sooner you get to experience life as a slimmer and happier you.

Many Blessings on your journey to a happier and slimmer you.

To Your Health,

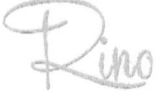

12 Weeks To A Healthy & Slim Body

Week 1

Setting The Holistic Foundation For Being Healthy and Slim

- Make The Decision To Change Your Life and Walk Your Talk

- Clean Out Your Cupboards and Pantry of Unhealthy Foods

- Begin Filling Your Pantry With Wholesome Ingredients From the Body Brilliance Grocery List

- When Dining Out, Follow The Body Brilliance Principles For Meal Selections

- When Grocery Shopping, Purchase Food Ingredients From The Body Brilliance Grocery List.

Ok my friend, the time has come for you to step up to the plate and begin your path a healthier and slimmer you. The pathway I have created is simple yet very powerful. The only thing required is for you to make the commitment to stay on path and do your daily practices that get results. If you can learn to embody what I am teaching here, you will have a solid foundation that will serve you the rest of your life. The results you get will change your life and they will last because you are embodying a holistic lifestyle that ensures ongoing results.

Ok, so in week 1 of your Body Brilliance Holistic Slimming Makeover your task is to reset your mind and view this as a mission that is Bigger than just you. If you can view this as a mission that will not only transform your life by becoming slim and healthy, but also that you will be helping the entire planet to evolve and transform as well.

A healthy and radiant society is conducive to True evolution and for creating harmony. Healthy and radiant people are kinder and gentler and have more love for people and the earth. When your body is functioning optimally, your emotions will be more balanced and you will feel more grounded.

Remember, that mind, body and spirit are all interconnected and what affects one of these affects the others just as a rock thrown into a pond ripples and affects the entire pond. So, your task for this first week is to simply adjust your thinking to reflect a Higher consciousness in that your level of health impacts the entire planet.

Also, please begin to say the following affirmation either out loud or quietly as much as possible. You will be surprised to how powerful this can be.

My Body Is A Sacred Temple & I Lovingly Take Care Of It!

Make this your mantra and feel the power of this simple affirmation. If you meditate then this is a good time for you to simply honor and appreciate your body for what is does for you. Your body is your main vehicle to experience this game of life, so begin to view it as a Sacred Vehicle that you love to take care of just as you would take care of a small child.

My revolutionary and proprietary *Body Brilliance Holistic Slimming Formula* for structuring meals is as follows: **For each main meal, you in**

essence have half of your plate be veggies, this includes raw or steamed or both.

The other half of your plate gets a half of protein serving as in meats, eggs, and cheese, **and the other half gets a complex carbohydrate** as in wild rice, brown rice, quinoa, sweet potato, millet and sprouted grain bread as in manna bread or gluten free bread. Also, be sure to eat 3 holistic meals per day as to ensure you are supplying your body with its requirements.

Be aware that if you eat infrequently or not enough for your body type, this will cause your body to go into survival mode which in turn then alters your basal metabolic rate to burn calories slower. Make sure to eat every 3 to 4 hours as to ensure your body stays in balance and your metabolism is at efficient levels. Also, include one piece of fruit per day, however, eat this in late afternoon about 2 hours before your dinner.

If you are going to do any desserts then do so 2 hours before dinner as well since this is best for your holistic slimming makeover results. Do not ever eat desserts after dinner as this is not ideal for digestion and for slimming results.

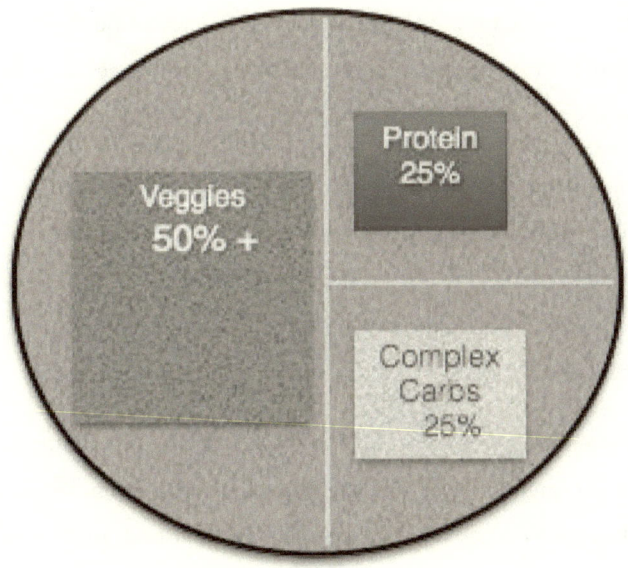

This is what I call **The Perfect Plate™**. It is essentially the most balanced and holistic process for staying healthy and keeping slim. By ensuring you ingest at least half of all your main meals as veggies, this will help to keep your system alkalized and regular. If you can do more than 50% of your meals as veggies then even better. My formula is universally effective in helping anyone to slim their body quickly as long as you remove the grunge foods and follows my 12 week holistic slimming makeover to the letter. **The main reason why this is so is because fiber from plants has miraculous effects on your system and allows you to stay balanced and regular. Fiber is the key to staying slim and energized.**

In fact, this is the way most humans are designed to ingest nutrition as this perfect ratio of nutrition (**50%, 25%, 25%**) intake validates itself with results that last. The only factor required is to add some fat as in grapeseed oil, olive oil, coconut oil, butter or palm oil to complete the perfect balance. You can drizzle the oil or slivers of butter on top of the veggies or wild rice or brown rice to enhance the flavor.

Also, for this first week of your Body Brilliance Makeover please clean out your cupboards and pantry of any product or ingredient that is not healthy. Simply put these items into a box and then donate them to local charities. Also, remove from your refrigerator any unhealthy and toxic compounds. These include mayonnaise, all sodas, all sugar products, all canned and processed foods.

The next thing you want to do is begin stocking your pantry and refrigerator with life giving foods and ingredients. **Items such as olives, fresh nuts, fresh organic vegetables, sprouted grain bread, gluten-free bread, organic pasture butter, goat yogurts, goat cheeses, gluten-free flours such as sorghum flour, brown rice flour, almond flour, coconut flour, wild rice, organic frozen veggie packs, quinoa, free range fatty portion meats, free range eggs, sea salt, organic spices.**

Holistic Tips For Dining Out

When dining out please use the following practices so that you may ensure you stay on path. Please understand that most restaurants use unhealthy ingredients in preparing their menu items so it is your duty to learn how to order to keep it clean and healthier.

You have a right to get menu items customized to your desire. Just because an item is on the menu does not mean you have to go with it. ASK! ASK! ASK! Ask for what you desire! For example, if you are going to order the house salad then make sure to tell them to leave off the dressing and instead bring you a small dish of olive oil that you will drizzle on.

You can also ask them for some lemon slices that you can squeeze on your salad as well. You can also request to have avocado slices added on your salad and things like walnuts and even feta cheese.

Stay away from corn chips as these are fried and toxic to your system, they are also GMO, most corn is GMO and not a healthy food item. Stay away from fried food items and anything dripping with sauces as these may contain MSG and other flavoring compounds in them. Stay away from all breads and white flour products as they are unhealthy and cause weight gain.

Also stay away from white rice as it is pure starch and can cause weight gain. Stay away from potatoes as they are super starchy and unhealthy since they are GMO (genetically modified).

Order items such as fresh guacamole, freshly made salsas, clean soups and similar items, Use veggie sticks to dip instead of chips and bread.

For main entrees, order items such as roasted chicken dishes, grilled salmon, rib eye steak well done – make sure to get red meat cooked well done as they have parasites in them and you require to cook at high heat to remove them.

Also you may order items such as grilled veggies and brown rice. Order extra sides of grilled veggies if you are hungry.

So, a sample meal that you can order at most restaurants is as follows:

Salad with avocado and walnuts with olive oil and lemon, a side of guacamole with veggie sticks and main entrée of half roasted chicken with brown rice and lots of extra grilled veggies. This is pretty clean and healthy and is a balanced meal.

When grocery shopping, I recommend following my **Body Brilliance Grocery List Guide** as it lists all of the main food ingredients that are super healthy and will help you to stay on path to a healthier and slimmer you.

Ok, this is more than enough for you to get rolling on for week 1 of your Body Brilliance Holistic Slimming Makeover. Do the best you can and make sure to chant your mantra as much as possible. You are also setting a foundation here in week one and it is very important to get your home structured so that it is easier to stay on path such as having clean foods in your refrigerator and pantry.

Week 2

Your Body Brilliance

- Your Body Is A Sacred Temple

- Caring For Your Sacred Temple

- What To Put In, On and Around Your Body Temple

- Your Body Temple Runs Via Energy and Is The Main Component To Your Health

- Your Body Temple Requires Maintenance

Ok, so for week 2 you are learning how to view your body as a Sacred Temple...because it is my friend. Your body is the most immaculate creation in the entire Universe. If you only knew just how amazing and brilliant your body is, you would marvel at its Divine Perfection.

You see, your body is not a machine that you can dump whatever you want into it. It is a living creation that requires specific types of compounds in order for it to function properly. Your body is performing billions of bio-chemical processes every second and it does so with complete consistency. Your body regenerates your entire physiology over and over again. Your body is truly an amazing creation and it is Divine. Every single cell in your body is alive and conscious and they are like little babies that requires your daily support.

You are the parent to billions of little babies that require nourishment and nurturing each day. Your cells are constantly looking for nourishment in the form of holistic nutrition and nurturing in the form of love. The time has come for you and the rest of humanity to view your body as a living conscious creation that you are responsible for. If you know that you are carrying billions of living babies with you, how will treat them?

Will you continue to dump grunge and toxic foods into your body? Or will you begin to input clean, healthy and holistic foods ingredients that will help your cell babies to thrive? This is a simple perspective change that can dramatically change your life. Please begin to view your body as a collective of billions of living babies that require you to be responsible and take care of them as you would a small child.

The mantra or affirmation for Week 2:

I Love My Cell Babies and Feed Them Healthy and Energizing Foods So They May Thrive

Look, everything you put in, on or around your body ought to be as clean and healthy as possible as this translates into your body being able to give you energy. **It is all about energy my friend.** Your nutrition gets converted into energy. If you have energy then you have life. If you have life then you can live life on a Higher plane. Most people do not have much energy because of the daily food choices they make. In turn, they do not have much life and thus cannot live fulfilled lives. Most people are ingesting compounds each day that actually take energy from the body so thus you have what you got and that is a depleted and overweight society.

Please begin to elevate your consciousness to view your health and your daily nutrition in the form of energy. The Higher the quality of your nutrition then the Higher levels of energy you will have and thus you then can experience life on a Higher plane of living. This is the most important component to health.

Be more conscious of what you are putting into your body and view it as qualities of energy. **Natural foods will supply you with high quality energy.** Processed foods, sugar and unnatural compounds will give you either low quality energy or actually take energy away from your body as do almost all processed sugar foods and drinks.

Be sure to also view that what you put on your body is also affecting your health. So, begin to throw out your body products as in shampoos, toothpaste, skin creams, makeups, perfumes, colognes and any other body product as these may contain many toxic ingredients in them. Begin to purchase natural and organic skin care products that are plant based and use natural essential oils. Your body shall thank you!

Week 3

The Multiple Dimensions of Your Health

- Your Level of Health is Determined By More Than Just Your Physical Nature

- The Holistic Wheel Of Life and Its Link To Your Health and Well Being

- How To Balance The Wheel of Life For Elevating Your Well Being

In week 3 of your Body Brilliance Holistic Slimming Makeover you are going to learn about the complete complex of who you are and what it requires to be optimally healthy. You are more than a physical body and more than you can see with your eyes. In fact, the physical aspect to your being is a small portion of the totality of you. You see, you are comprised of a mental, emotional and spiritual aspect as well or what some call soul. So, our modern society has gotten way off path of this Truth and has reduced people to just bodies and physicality. No mystery as to why so many people are not healthy and slim these days. Just in case you do not know the Truth...is that you are 90% spiritual and only 10% physical.

Also, your mental, emotional and spiritual complex have more of a pull on your health than do physical factors alone. In fact, your level of health is determined by at least 80% of how well balanced you are in these unseen aspects to your being.

The time has come for you and humanity to elevate your consciousness to see the Truth that you are multi-dimensional and require nourishing the unseen aspects to your being as well if you desire to be optimally healthy. I have created a simple model that will help you to see the Truth of how important it really is to be balanced in your entire physical, mental, emotional and spiritual complex.

So, if you will picture a large round wheel with a smaller circle inside. You then have a wheel with four quadrants and an inner circle like the graphic shown.

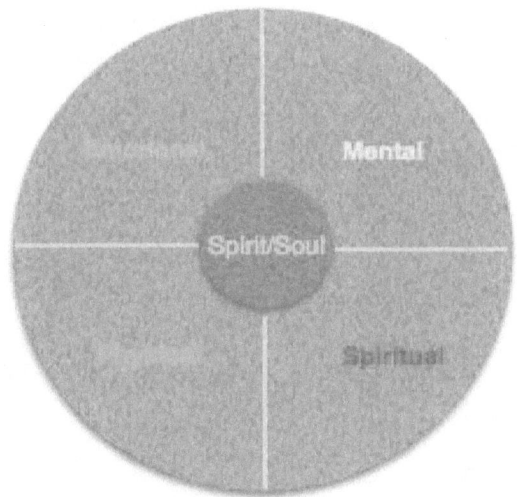

This is your Wheel of Life and is the key for you being able to experience optimum health and well-being and for evolving your spirit.

This is your wheel of life. Think of it as you sitting inside your car ready to drive into the world. Now, in order for you to have a smooth ride in life and to have your steering be straight, you require all 4 aspects of your being balanced. Do you get this? Your emotional, mental, physical and spiritual complex requires to be in harmony, integrated and balanced for you to have a life that flows, feels good and is expansive.

Now, picture if you had only 1 tire inflated properly on your car and the other 3 inflated at different capacities. Or picture if you have one flat tire. Do you think you can drive anywhere with a flat tire? How about having 2 flat tires? Are you going anywhere my friend? And then what about having 3 flat tires or all 4 tires flat? My point is you require all 4 tires balanced and inflated properly to be able to drive straight and go anywhere.

Here is a reality check for you and humanity just to see where we are at as a totality consciousness attempting to go somewhere in this life. Most of humanity is attempting to go through life with only 1 aspect of their life intact and even that aspect is unbalanced. Most humans are only looking at one aspect to their being which is physical. And...the process they are using to physical health is way off and most aren't even coming near what is required physically to attain and maintain their health.

My friend, most of humanity is attempting to drive through life with only one wheel in life and that wheel is flat because they are using information that is erroneous to say least.

Most people do not know that it is a requirement of your health to nourish your mental, emotional and spiritual complex. Most people do not know about holistic nutrition and how to truly nourish their body. Do you see this? Do you see why our society has millions of people who are overweight and unhealthy? Do you see why so many people have life issues? You get it now, right?

In order for you to be absolutely healthy, slim and radiant, you require to balance your wheel of life. It is the only way you can be healthy and live a fulfilled life. You must learn how to nourish all aspects of your being. This is vital to not only your physical health, it is also the only way to your evolution as a human being.

Does this resonate with you? Are you beginning to have an understanding of what health really is? This is absolutely the key to your health and living your most victorious life.

In essence, for your **True Self/Spirit** to carry you through life and help you to evolve, you require a wheel of life that is balanced in your physical, mental, emotional and spiritual complex. It is like having a car that is aligned properly and has 4 tires inflated to ideal measures. In this level of harmony and balance, now you get to experience life on a much Higher level as your **True Self/Spirit** can drive you to many expansive horizons.

Balancing Your Wheel Of Life

In order for you to balance and harmonize your Wheel of Life, you require elevating your consciousness to see that you are a multi-dimensional being. You require nourishing your full being of mind, body and spirit. You do this by taking some time each day and sitting with yourself and simply connecting with these parts to you.

You sit quietly and begin to feel your inner components of who you truly are. You begin to connect with them by simply placing your consciousness on them. You may even speak out loud and begin to dialogue with these aspects of your being. You may also chant and sing or whatever comes naturally. Ask that you be forgiven for not honoring and nourishing these aspects to your being. Show sincerity that you are going to honor and nourish them from now on and ask what it is you can do to help balance your Wheel of Life.

I recommend going out in nature for hikes and walks as nature is conscious and Mother Earth will help you to restore your full being if you simply ask. Look, this inner process is more important to your well-being than anything else in life. You will feel shifts if you are willing to do the inner process of balancing and harmonizing yourself.

Your affirmation for week 3 is:

I Love My Mind, Body and Spirit & Lovingly Nourish Them

Week 4

Holy Water, Sacred Water

The Key For Experiencing Higher Levels of Health

- Water Is The Key Compound For Creating Optimum Health

- Properly Structured Water Is Essential For Being Healthy, Slim and Radiant

- How To Create Properly Structured Water

Ok, so in Week 4 of your Body Brilliance Holistic Makeover, you are going to learn more about water and why it is the catalyst to helping you for slimming yourself down naturally and holistically. You will also discover how water is the link to your evolution and living your most victorious life. I already talked about water in a previous chapter, however, I want to remind you of some very important factors to water and how it is the compound that can make everything else you do for health work better and more efficiently.

Essentially, water is the most Sacred compound in the entire Universe. There are many qualities to water that are so amazing and some indigenous cultures have known for some time how Divine this compound really is. There are many factors at play with water that if you can learn may dramatically shift your life in profound ways.

Water is the main vehicle or mechanism that your body requires to transport bio-nutrients to and from where they are supposed to go. Water is also the main cleanser of your body as it helps to expel bio-wastes and other toxins out through your elimination channels. As I spoke about in a previous chapter there is an issue with the water of today as the molecular structure has been altered from its Divine state. As such, water is not able to do what it is supposed to do in helping you to be healthy and cleansed.

You see, water is the key compound and link to your evolution as a human being. Your brain is the master computer and link into your Higher faculties. Essentially, your brain requires lots of water along with key bio-nutrients to be able to process upper dimensional information and frequencies that you require to be healthy and for your evolution.

If your brain does not receive adequate quantities of hydration each day then your Higher faculties cannot be activated and thus you will experience a limited life as your Higher gifts and talents will not be able to come through.

Many gifted people like musicians and artists have their unique talents because their brain is pulling in Higher dimensional information that allows them to be so. So, if you want to experience a super healthy and expansive life you will require hydrating your body properly each day. Hydrating water will impact your life on all levels of mind, body and soul. Water affects your body by transporting nutrients to where they are supposed to and also by detoxing bio-wastes and other toxins.

Water affects you emotionally as well because a fully hydrated and clean body automatically translates into feeling better. Water will also affect you at the soul level as your radiant health and brain hydration will allow you to tap into your Higher Potentials that translates into you being able to express your unique gifts and talents.

As you can see, water is a Sacred gift of the Divine Creator and you ought to learn more about it as there is a reason why water has always been revered as Holy or Sacred in many traditions on planet Earth throughout history. There is a reason why most of humanity lives and has lived very near bodies of water. In fact, at least 3/4 of the earth's population currently lives by water. There is a reason why almost every single person loves being at the beach and lakes and streams.

People can feel the resonance of water and unconsciously know that it is healthy to be around. Water is the main vehicle of life and for evolution as a species and for planet earth. Even animals seem to know how Sacred water is as they usually congregate and live near waterways of planet earth.

Are you beginning to view water as more than just an aqueous compound that hydrates? Are you feeling a shift in your being in regards to how amazing water is? Do you see the Truth of the importance of water for health and evolution for all life on planet earth? Wouldn't you think that it should be the most important aspect to life and that we as a humanity ought to revere it more than it is currently? Don't you think you as a human who cares for your life and your evolution, ought to know more of how to truly hydrate your body and the Divine qualities to water?

Well, I will help you now to learn more about how to structure water for better hydration. As I spoke about in a previous chapter, most bottled water is not healthy to consume and in fact can be quite acidic. You can validate this for yourself by simply getting some litmus paper and dipping into any bottled water. You will discover that most bottled waters will show they are acidic.

Filtering water changes the molecular structure and can also make it acidic as do reverse osmosis and distillation. There are also other water purification systems that can make water unhealthy to drink as in deionization and essentially any process where you are filtering or changing the molecular structure of water.

So, the easiest and most efficient way to help transform your water to be more hydrating and healthier is to bless your water or pray over it. There is a reason why Holy Water has been known to help some people to heal health conditions. You see, Holy Water is water that has been blessed by a spiritual person with prayers of the Creator. These prayers get imbued into the water and the water shifts the molecules to reflect what the prayer says. This may sound way out there, however, it is of Truth.

You can view the books by Dr. Masaru Emotto as he clearly shows scientifically how water can be changed at the molecular level by simply praying over it or by placing photos of beauty and harmony under a glass of water.

You can begin to do your own experiments with this simple process of blessing your water and see the Truth. Simply take a glass of water, place your hands around it and call in God, Source, Holy Spirit or whatever you call your Higher Power and ask for the water to be blessed for your body and radiant health. *You can also send the following affirmation into the glass yourself:* **I Love You Water and You Now Hydrate My Body Optimally. You Are Pure, You Are Divine, You Are Sacred! Thank You**

Begin drinking this water every day and notice any shifts in your health or body or even your emotions. Make sure to bless your water each time you drink. This is a very simple process and very cost effective.

You can feed your plants some of this water as plants are super conscious by the way and will quickly reveal to you if water is good or not. Give your plants this Holy Water for a week and watch what happens to them. Give it a try and let life show you Truth.

There is also a device that I have discovered that works to restructure water naturally and holistically. Essentially, this device helps water to remember its Sacred Structuring and the results speak for themselves. I have also created a product called Aqua Light that is out of this world super charged for hydration. If you will like more information simply visit my website and check out:

www.rinosoriano.com

Week 5

Full Body Cleansing

The Catalyst For Holistic Slimming and Being Radiant

- The Truth About Cleansing

- Why You Need To Cleanse Your Body Right Now

- Cleansing Your Body Properly

- How To Cleanse Your Sacred Temple Effectively and Efficiently

Ok, this is week 5 of your Body Brilliance Holistic Slimming Makeover and so now that you are on roll with eating cleaner and hydrating your body better, the time is now for you to begin to cleanse your body of heavy metals, parasites and bio-wastes that have accumulated over time.

Be aware that there are many detox kits out there nowadays and I will say that most of these kits are not going to be able to cleanse your body of years' worth of accumulated toxicities and parasites. The 3, 5 and 7 day detox kits simply will not be able to purge these out since you require the proper hydration and also the proper supplements that will begin to activate your detox channels.

There are specific compounds that will help to activate your body's natural enzyme system and also other bodily detox mechanisms. You require learning what these compounds are and how to use them properly. The key is to keep it efficient and cost effective. Your body does not want many supplements thrown at it and ones that simply cannot do what is being claimed.

Also, most supplements can actually be a pollutant to your body as many companies add fillers, binders and other compounds that literally make them toxic to your system. So, the key factor is for you to learn how to cleanse your body properly and keep it cost effective and efficient. This is something you learn through one on one coaching and is a service I do for people because it is important to learn how to do this holistically. If you go at this detox process yourself, you will waste time, money and energy and you may actually mess up your up health as some people have done by wanting to explore and experiment on their own.

Do yourself a favor and invest in this service and learn a simple and holistic process for cleansing. This is much simpler than it may sound and when you take the proper supplements then the results are profound. So, keep it simple and cost effective. I can show you how to do this for yourself and help you to support your system as to help expel toxicities efficiently.

You will be surprised at how amazing you begin to feel as you clear out toxins, parasites and yeast from your body. You will feel as if a new life has been granted to you. You see, all the toxicities, parasites and yeast put a load on your system and rob you of pure energy. They make your body function inefficiently and this translates into a lack of energy and vitality.

As you begin to clear these things out, your body now has the energy to function properly and to help you feel well. You will notice that your skin health will improve and the texture of your hair as now your liver can do it functions. You may even notice your mood is better and that you are calmer.

You may also notice that you feel more joyful and that you want to go out and do great things. You may want to sing or dance or just celebrate how you feel.

This is supposed to be natural and how all humans ought to feel and be like each day. However, with our toxic modern society, this is no longer the case so you require walking the holistic pathway to attain this level of health. Then once you attain optimum health, you require maintaining it consistently by keep walking the holistic path.

The holistic pathway helps you to attain radiant health and then maintain it. This now becomes a lifestyle that keeps getting you results because you are embodying natural and holistic principles for optimum health. This is very simple and yet very profound.

Most health paradigms out there are not teaching holistic principles for optimum health. They are teaching erroneous myths that do not validate themselves and do not give people lasting results. I am teaching you a holistic pathway that honors your body, mind and spirit and how they are supposed to be treated, nourished and nurtured as to provide the best process for helping you to be healthy, slim and radiant.

Keep walking the path my friend, you will see and feel many beautiful shifts in your body and your life as you do. For now you can go **www.rino-soriano.com/body-brilliance-detox-kit/** to get my Body Brilliance Detox Remedies for free and begin with that.

Your affirmation for the week is:

I Love My Body & It Now Rejuvenates Itself Back To Its Sacred Perfection

Week 6

Ground Thyself

- **What Is Natural Grounding**

- **Why You Require To Ground Yourself Consistently**

- **How To Ground Yourself Properly**

- **Grounding Is Your Direct Link To Your Higher Expression and To Source**

Here you are at week 6 of your life transforming journey. How are you doing? Do you feel big shifts in your consciousness and your health? Keep on path as you will be taking a few big steps in the next few weeks that may super charge your holistic slimming results.

Ok, so today you are going to learn about natural grounding and how it is an essential component to your health. Most people simply do not know about this simple yet profound holistic health elixir of life. In fact, natural grounding is as important as nutrition yet not many people are talking about this or know the profundity of what this can do for your health and wellness levels.

So, what is natural grounding? Grounding is literally connecting to Mother Earth in some way as in having your bare feet or butt-i-simo on terra-firma. This means to have a part of your bare body to actually touch the earth in some way. This act literally grounds you and provides you an opportunity to have one of the greatest influxes of earth energy. It is an all body elixir and can dramatically elevate your health levels in quantum leaps.

You see, Mother Earth is one BIG electro-magnetic generator of grounding energy. Your body requires this earth energy to be balanced and healthy. There is a reason why all of the Indigenous cultures to ever walk this planet lived in tribes and low to the ground. They knew that Mother Earth is our life line to life and our health so they built their home structures low to earth and so ensuring they were always connected. This earth energy is the greatest remedy for you and your body.

By grounding consistently, you take in this healing energy as to give your body a boost and a charge of pure life force power. The Hawaiians call it Manna, the East Indians call it Prana, the Asians call it Chi. Essentially, it is pure life force energy that animates everything in the entire Universe. It gives flowers their life force to be flowers and it helps animals to be animals and for you to be you.

Our society has as a whole has most people who lack life force energy because they do not go out in nature to ground on a consistent basis. As such, their health levels and their overall energy level is low. The modern society has pulled people off path from this natural health remedy by making life about man-made structures and superficial ways of living. So, thus you get what you got and that is a society that is very depleted of life force energy. You need this life force energy to be able to experience life on a High level and for your evolution. It has many qualities that go beyond physical well-being benefits. Grounding and the life force energy you pull in from Mother Earth can elevate your consciousness by giving you a link to the consciousness of the planet.

Accessing earth's consciousness via grounding will provide you a catapult in your evolution as you can learn about profound life wisdom by simply being connected to Mother Earth. This is how all of the indigenous cultures were and are so wise. They knew how to tap into the consciousness of Mother Earth and learn many profound Truths about nature, the earth and the Universe.

You see, by being connected and grounded to Mother Earth, it links you to Universal Consciousness. Do you understand now why being grounded is so important to your health and evolution? It is your direct link to accessing the grand Universal Bank of wisdom and knowledge of all life. It is powerful because you can learn more about life and the Universe in a few days than you have ever learned in your entire life. And...the information that you have learned in schools and academia is a pure pittance compared to what you will learn from Mamma Earth.

She is the grand teacher of us all and she teaches Truth, not theories and funny paradigms as society has done with man-made philosophies. Thus, you have a society that is limited in what it can create and achieve. Society has become a hodge-podge of superficiality that does not nourish the body let alone the spirit.

So, if you really care for your health and well-being and for your evolution while you are on this Sacred planet, then it will be wise for you to begin natural grounding practices and feel the shifts in your body and life. Essentially, you go out in nature somewhere, it can be a park with grass, a field, a forest, a beach, a mountain or dessert and you touch Mamma Earth with either your bare feet or you sit your butt-i-simo on the ground. You can use this time to simply just connect with nature and Mother Earth. Appreciate nature for it is so beautiful. Observe the animals, the sunshine, the clouds, the wind blowing the trees and flowers. Breathe deeply and pull in fresh air. Visualize yourself having energy roots coming from your feet and butt going down into Mother Earth.

Now after you have rooted yourself in the ground, you can then begin to visualize pulling up white life force energy from Mother Earth and see it bathe and nourish your entire body. You will be amazed at how great you feel by making this a consistent practice you do a few times a week. If you can do more than a few times a week or every day then go for it as you will feel and see the effects.

Be aware that our society is way off path from our natural Divine blueprint for health. Everything in life has become synthetic and man-made from your home, to your clothes, to even the food supply. My friend, you cannot sustain life for long on synthetic living. Of all things you learn in my teachings, please know this...**that you require life force energy to have health, to have a family, to have a business, to live life.**

How can you live life to the fullest if you do not have life force energy? You may think right now that you have energy...well, my friend...what you have is a stimulated system that is running on false energy. If the food supply you are ingesting has no life giving energy in it, if your home is made of synthetic compounds (which all homes do in modern society), if your car is synthetic, your place of work is synthetic and your clothes are synthetic then where are you getting energy from?

You can only get this life force energy from nature and from foods that are heirloom and unaltered (80% of the food supply is either hybridized or

GMO at this point), from clothing materials that are natural, from a home that is made from natural earth materials and from a career that makes your heart sing. So, do you really think you have pure energy at this point? Do you think you can continue this hamster wheel lifestyle for much longer?

My main teaching here is about energy and your health is about the accretion and accumulation of life force energy. This is the most important aspect to your health that you require learning. When you have pure life force energy animating your body, you will feel it and so will others around you.

It is very powerful. Not many people in society have True life force energy because they do not know the practices of how to take in life force energy and maintain it. So, if you want to be healthy and live an extended life then you may want to learn more about grounding and other practices that help you to accumulate this powerful life force energy. You may contact me if you want to learn about my services about other natural life force building practices.

The affirmation for this week is

I Now Ground Myself To My Source Of Life Force Energy. I Easily Accumulate Life Force Energy in My Body and I Am Naturally Energized! Thank you Mother Earth, You Are So Beautiful!

Week 7

Holistic Fitness

A Holistic Path For Being Slim, Tone and Energized

- What Is Holistic Fitness?

- Fun Fitness That You Love To Do

- How To Do Holistic Fitness That Gets Results For Being Healthy, Slim and Energized

Ok, in week 7 of your super holistic slimming journey I am going to teach you about holistic fitness. I spoke about holistic fitness a bit in a previous chapter and so I will expand on why holistic fitness is the most efficient practice for getting fit and slim. As I said in the previous chapter, most fitness practices being taught out there are not efficient or wise for long term health benefits. Some fitness activities are actually depleting to your system and some quite unhealthy.

I teach holistic fitness practices that honor the nature of your body and get results that last. Once again, it is about energy my friend. You want to conserve energy when you do any activity or sport, so thus the holistic fitness I teach helps you to conserve energy while benefitting your health and fitness gains.

Holistic fitness is essentially performing fitness activities that help your body to get tone and fit while elevating your health levels. Holistic fitness honors your body and the way it is designed so thus you experience results much faster and you will see that they last.

Your body requires to be worked out in a holistic manner and in fact you will be quite surprised at how this process for getting fit and slim is much easier on your physiology. You actually enjoy engaging in holistic fitness because it is energizing and uplifting to your inner being as well. You only require minimal time and moderate efforts to get results.

So, how do you go about holistic fitness and what makes it so effective? Well, first off is that it will conserve you lots of energy because you will be focusing on activities and sports that actually build your energy reserves. Most types of fitness and sports are depleting to your system as they consume too much energy and deplete your nutrient reserves.

Sweating causes you to deplete your nutrient reserves and most people do not know how to replenish them properly. This sets you up for becoming very deficient in key bio-nutrients. Activities like running, marathons, cardio aerobics, treadmill and other such activities where you are expending lots of energy and sweating will deplete your system and cause low level health eventually.

So, in performing holistic fitness you are building energy and conserving your nutrient reserves. This is life enhancing and will serve to also help get you get slim and fit in record time. The most effective means of getting fit and tone quickly is to engage in activities that incorporate the use of your muscles without taxing your cardiovascular and nutrient reserve systems. Activities such as hiking, power walking, pilates, tennis, volleyball, power yoga and weight training are the best means of fitness as they conserve energy and bio-nutrients as you will not be sweating profusely as you will with other sports and activities.

I feel that weight training in a holistic manner is the greatest means of getting tone and for extending your life. When you work out in this holistic manner, you help your body to produce many life enhancing hormones such as hGH which is the hormone that can help keep you young and healthy. It has many rejuvenating qualities and has been show to increase in production in your body when you perform the proper weight training.

When doing holistic weight training, you will only be working out for 30 minutes or less. Essentially, you will be doing high intensity movements for short duration and thus you will conserve energy. For example, if you are working out your biceps, you will do a set and only rest for like 5 seconds. You then pick up the next heavier weight and do another set. You rest 5 seconds only again and pick up the next heavier weight and do another set.

You do this for like 5 minutes straight. You will see that your muscles are pumped and yet you have conserved lots of energy in the process. It is like condensing a 30 minute body part work out session into 5 minutes.

This is super-efficient and is the most ideal form of training that your muscles benefit the most from. Your muscles want to be worked out as hard as possible in the shortest amount of time possible. Your muscles only have so much ATP and nutrient reserves to be in anabolic phase while you work out. So, most people are doing themselves a disservice by working out for an hour and spending large amounts of time doing one body part. You do not require working out a body part for that long.

Hiking is another great life enhancing activity that elevates your energy levels and can also be grounding and provide emotional and mental benefits as well. Hiking helps many muscles in your body to get worked out in optimal fashion while conserving energy and bio-nutrients.

Hiking is like an all body workout while keeping your system optimized and conserving energy. Hiking is fun and you also get to benefit from receiving sunlight for optimum health. Hiking can also be used as a daily grounding activity after you come home and are looking to calm your physiology. Hiking can do wonders to help calm your emotions and balance your mood.

If you are looking to get into really good shape really fast then you can put on a back pack with weight in it of some kind like water bottles, bricks, books or any object with weight and go power walking. You can increase the weight you put in your backpack every week or 2 to provide more endurance and stimulation to your body and muscles as to help you get tone while helping you to shed body weight.

Another holistic secret for getting tone and fit quickly is by using ankle and wrist weights while hiking or simply walking. You can also wear these throughout the day under you clothes while you work, while you shop, while you do the laundry or anytime where you will be walking or doing home activities. This is a fantastic way of getting in shape while conserving energy and shedding the weight. Give it a try and see.

My recommendation is for you to do at least 3 days a week of some kind of holistic fitness activity I just revealed. If you work out with weights then you can do an entire body workout in 30 minutes or less as I detailed earlier. Simply go through each body part and take like 5 minutes to do as many sets as possible or when your body part says it has had enough.

Your affirmation for the week is:

My Body Is Getting Fit & Tone and I Love Doing My Holistic Fitness

Week 8

Healthy Hobbies

- Healthy Hobbies Can Transform Your Life

- How Healthy Hobbies Elevate Your Health Levels

- Healthy Hobbies Keep You Balanced and Happy

In week 8 you are going to learn about how having healthy hobbies that make your heart sing can actually improve your health and well-being. Hobbies are an integral part of helping you to balance your life and to expand your boundaries. Hobbies offer you an opportunity to elevate your health levels and to connect with other people of like mind interested in the same activities.

Anytime you do an activity that makes you happy or gives you a sense of belonging, it actually causes your body to produce many life enhancing bio-chemicals that elevate your health and well-being. This is something that you can feel pretty distinctly if you simply get more in tune with your body.

You see, at the fundamental level of your health, there is a direct connection to your brain and the unique array of neurotransmitters and hormones that get produced with each emotion and activity that you experience.

If you really become conscious of your life, then you will begin to notice that you get specific feelings with each life event that you experience. As such, your body then produces a unique elixir of neurons and hormones that directly affects how you feel.

Having hobbies and other activities such as recreational sports gives your body a boost of life force energy and also helps to calm your physiology as it directly affects your brain and its balancing. You see, you have 2 hemispheres to your brain and when you engage in hobbies and sports it temporarily synchronizes both brain hemispheres to act as one unit.

This synergizing process has many life giving benefits to your health and body. Again, this is something you can feel and experience if you are in tune with your body.

It is a wise practice to have hobbies in your life that make your heart sing. They are essential to your health and psychology and for living a balanced life. You require healthy hobbies for also connecting with other people as to help you be more social.

Being social and connecting with others can also have an effect on your health and well-being. Once again, you brain will produce many life enhancing bio-chemicals from the interaction with other people, especially if you have love for them. It has been shown scientifically that people who are part of a group of some kind have better health and well-being than people who tend to do things alone or never really go out and do much.

It has also been shown that people who have pets usually have better health than people who do not. Again, this is due to your brain producing a bio-chemical elixir that raises the frequency of your body. The secret is that it is LOVE that keeps the body healthy and strong. If you have love for people and pets then your level of health seems to be much higher than if you do not have much love for life as a whole.

So, my main teaching for now is be involved in hobbies that make your heart sing as it will catapult your health and well-being. Be part of a group of people that you love to be with. Start your own group if you do not know of any. Just get out and explore with hobbies and groups of various kinds and you will feel and see shifts in your health. Be sure to make hobbies, sports and group activities an integral part of your holistic health pathway, as to do so will catapult your evolution as a human being. Happy Hobbies!!!

Your affirmation for this week is:

I Love My Hobbies and Sports As They Make My Body Happy and Healthy

Week 9

Mind Detox

Subconscious Deprogramming and Reprogramming

- What Is A Mind Detox

- How To Clear Limiting Beliefs and Programs

- How To Reprogram Yourself For Higher Potentials

- Embracing Your Magnificent Self To Serve Your Life Mission

Ok, are you ready for the next catapult on your holistic health makeover journey? This week you are going to learn how to begin detoxing your mind of outdated beliefs, erroneous myths and misinformation that are keeping you on the hamster wheel of life. You require purging all of the limiting beliefs, attitudes and philosophies that you have been conditioned with since your birth if you truly desire to evolve your soul. This is one of the most essential processes you require on your holistic makeover journey as to do so will dramatically catapult your health and wellness and your entire life for that matter.

Your beliefs are nothing other than a certain statement about life that you think is true. Your beliefs about life and specific topics can cause you to experience many limiting events in your life. Your beliefs can be a hindrance to your evolution and also your health. Just so you know is that a belief does not necessarily mean that what you believe is absolutely true.

In fact, in our modern society there is a mountain of information out there being taught as truth which then programs people to believe it to be so. In fact, if you do a little exploring, you will come to discover that most information in society is limiting and in some cases quite harmful to your health and well-being. My teachings expose a lot of the grunge information out there for what it is. I keep things simple and use life and experience to validate if something is true or not. This is quite simple yet most people fall for the hype and misinformation and thus it becomes their beliefs which they think are true when they are not.

I have clearly clarified for you throughout my book here how there are so many myths and erroneous philosophies out there that simply do not validate themselves. The issue is because you have been programmed to believe certain things, your beliefs serve as programs that run on autopilot and limit your expression in life.

You have to understand that the Universe will mirror to you what you maintain in consciousness in the form of beliefs and feelings about certain topics of life. So, if you believe something to be True then you can be certain that the Universe will eventually mirror this belief to you in the form of life events somehow.

Now here is where things can get funny because beliefs can make your life more challenging and may cause you low level health. For example, before reading this book, you probably had the belief that it is healthy to limit your fat and calorie intake each day as to help you stay slim.

Well, as I revealed earlier, this common belief of limiting your fat and calories to get slim is erroneous. This myth has actually caused more people to gain excess weight overall because to follow this funny dietary practice will cause your body to go into survival mode and alter your metabolism to burn calories slower.

Some people have followed that erroneous myth for years and have not gotten any slimmer and some have even become heavier, yet they continue to follow that practice. This is the main issue with beliefs, they cause you to do things that may not be healthy or wise and in this case they will cause you to follow practices that are not conducive to helping you slim your body. Do you see this now? You require becoming conscious of your beliefs and begin to detox your mind of all erroneous philosophies and misinformation if you want radiant health and you desire to evolve yourself.

This is a requirement on your spiritual journey and is the only way to elevate your health and your consciousness for Higher Potentials in your life.

If we as a humanity are going to do anything productive as a species then we require to elevate our consciousness and shed outdated beliefs, erroneous philosophies and myth paradigms that stifle our evolution as is the case today on our planet.

Simply look at the current state of our planet and there you have a direct reflection of what kind of mind sets and beliefs humanity has created. This level of consciousness is parasitic and the Truth is there for you to see if you have the eyes to do so. Beliefs are a hindrance to health expansion and evolution and require to be shed. Beliefs are the cause of so much disharmony on this planet and have been so for thousands of years.

Beliefs are illusions people accept as Truth, yet they are false and have no substance other than the disharmony and disequilibrium they cause to all life on this Sacred jewel of a planet.

What we require as a collective is to simply follow nature and the Universal Laws that govern this expansive Universe. Now you may thinking, how can you live life without having beliefs? Actually, if humanity could purge and detox all of their beliefs at once, we would finally be able to create harmony and a paradise of this planet.

However, due to people loving to have belief systems, you have what you got today on this planet with disharmony and separation. With no beliefs we could easily create harmony because there would be no guards up from anyone and we would simply follow Truth of the Creator.

For example, the Truth that the sun rises in the east and sets in the west every day is a Universal Truth. It is so because you can validate this Truth every day with simple science and common sense. You do not need to believe that the sun rises in east and sets in the west.

My point is if we could simply learn to study life and follow its natural laws then we would not require any beliefs because we would simply be using Universal Truths to live by. No beliefs or philosophies are needed when you honor nature and follow its validation. Life and nature validate themselves with simple observance.

Beliefs are man-made philosophies that usually are not based on Absolute Truth. They are more of opinions than anything else. Life only reveals Truth if you have the eyes to see.

Getting rid of beliefs is the greatest gift that we can give this planet as Mother Earth has had enough of humanity's ignorance and inebriation with three dimensional thrills at the price of the planet and our well-being. Our modern society has become a superficial web of material priorities with total disregard for human life and for nature.

Our material world that has been created is toxic and parasitic to the planet and to us. Mother Earth is our life line and it does not make any sense on any level to strip and trash your home in order to satisfy human desires. At some point there is going to be a correction and maybe then humanity will be open to shedding its belief systems.

As you see beliefs cause disharmony and separation and are an impediment to human evolution. If you care for your health and the future of this planet, please for the sake of all humanity and Mother Earth begin to detox your mind of all belief systems you have. Many of these beliefs have been passed onto you by your family and others by society.

Trust me, you do not need your beliefs any longer as they will only serve to keep you on the hamster wheel of life that has no destination other than disharmony and a life of wasted energy.

Do you really want to maintain your beliefs? Please my friend, begin to shed these illusions as they are stifling to your Sacred Being and toxic to Mother Earth. You can shed them easily when you realize that life is about expression, exploration and LOVE.

You are here to express yourself and your unique talents, you are here to explore new horizons by learning new Truths about life and nature and you are here to LOVE with all your heart because that is what you really are.

You simply require waking up from your sleep and begin to view life in a new perspective. Life is meant to be lived as an adventure with each day like a blank canvas waiting for you to be the artist and create each day anew. Do you really want to continue your mundane life and being on the hamster wheel? Or do you want to be like a cosmic artist that gets to create a beautiful tapestry each day with your creative expression?

Let go of your beliefs and elevate your consciousness to begin arising from the grunge that you have allowed in your life. Detox your mind, your beliefs and your opinions of everything and allow life to reveal a new brilliant world where it is an adventure to behold each day. This reality exists already, you just have to shed the illusions that are preventing you from seeing it. They are your beliefs.

You begin shedding your beliefs by becoming conscious of every time you have an opinion about something. Behind that opinion you will find a belief system there. You may have thousands of beliefs systems about every topic of life. These beliefs systems are clouding your vision of what you think you see in the world.

Beliefs systems are like wearing colored glasses and will cause you to see a distorted vision of life. Simply begin by observing your thoughts on specific topics of when you have a conversation with someone. You will see just how many beliefs you have if you maintain conscious awareness of your conversation.

Almost every single statement you say is a belief or an opinion which has a belief system behind it. This is why this life has become so complex because you have billions of people with their own belief systems and each person is believing that the world is the way they see it. They are correct on one level, however, they are completely off on another level as it is their distorted belief system that is causing them to see the world the way they think it is. It is as they believe, not what the True reality of life actually is.

Life is a cosmic dance of constant change and expansion. Beliefs are fixed and limiting and do not take into account the Truth that life is constantly evolving.

To have beliefs is like trying to force life to stay still and be constant and never changing. That is not the way the Universe functions. In fact, the Universe is constantly changing and evolving to greater and more expansive expressions.

So, for you to have any beliefs, you are trying to go against what nature is about. You are attempting to keep life and nature constant and never changing. This is an impossibility as life is all about change and constant movement. Are you beginning to see how stifling belief systems really are? They are an impediment to life and to your evolution. Life is meant to be lived as an adventure where each day is like a new discovery of beauty.

If you have beliefs then it is like watching the same tv show episode over and over again every single day of your life. Do you think that would be fun? Do you think you could expand yourself and evolve your life in this manner?

This is why humanity does not see the inebriation with belief systems, because they are subtle and yet they cloud your vision of the world that is ever changing.

With beliefs, you can have no forward motion with your evolution as they are a fixed program or set of programs that are rigid and do not allow you to proceed. It is like having your car in park mode when you are attempting to drive down the street. Beliefs are like the parking gear that will not allow you to move forward and evolve. Beliefs are fixed illusions that appear to be real, however, they only have power because of your belief in them. Does this make sense? Does this resonate with you?

You can begin to remove your parking brakes by simply observing your language and thoughts and then begin to shed the opinions and statements that you think and say in your daily life. Learn to simply observe life and state Universal Truths that nature validates with experience.

Life will always reveal the Truth to you if you have the eyes to see. Begin to let life be your teacher of Universal Truths and you will see a whole new world and reality open up to you. Begin to affirm out loud these Universal Truths as you discover them. Affirm positive life statements that are uplifting and empowering. When in conversation with others be more conscious of your vocabulary and be the one who steers the topics to ones that are about the spiritual aspect to life, nature, animals and holistic health.

Your affirmation for this week is:

I Now Easily Shed My Beliefs As They Are Illusions. I Now Choose A Higher Reality Of Expression, Expansion and Love. I Love My New Life!

Week 10

Detoxing Your Entire Life

- The Importance Of Detoxing All Things In Your Life That Don't Support Your New Life

- How To Begin To Detox Your Life For Elevated Levels of Well Being

- Setting A New Foundation For Your Life That Supports Your New Holistic Lifestyle

How are you making out on your holistic health makeover journey? Are you experiencing quantum shifts and improvements in your health and well-being. Well, if you have been keeping on path of what I have been teaching you I think by now you are doing quite well.

This week is about setting a foundation for your entire life in the form of detoxing anything and everything that is not conducive for your expansion and well-being. This means it is time for you to shed people, places and things that are not high frequency or places that will pull your frequency down. It is about getting rid of material objects that you have no use for but just sit there and take up space.. In essence, this week 10 you are doing a complete life detox by removing any and all things that will pull you down in any way.

This may be the most challenging process for you as it will require you letting go of many attachments that are actually stifling to your evolution. You require doing this life detox because otherwise, these toxic attachments will serve to pull you off path at some point.

It is not easy to let go of people attachments, however, it is essential at times in your life to let go of friends and other people you routinely spend time with. What you want to do with this life detox is literally remove anyone or anything that is not on the same path as you.

You may view this as not proper to let go of a friend you have been spending time with for years, however, if they are living a toxic life and you spend time with them, they will eventually influence you to pull you off the holistic path. If you slip and fall off path then it will be much harder to get going again.

Do not allow this to happen. You may notice resistance coming in as you do this life detox because it means letting go of everything that you have used to feel safe and good.

This life detox will challenge you because it is literally causing you to be in your uncomfortable zone. However, this is the only way to get results with your slimming efforts and your evolution. At some point you have to go this route, otherwise, you will not be able to live a fulfilling life or tap into your Higher Potentials.

You probably also have many material objects that have been sitting around for years as do many people in society. You may think that some of these objects carry sentimental value so thus you save them. Well, if I may present a new perspective on this life detox process? Look, life is meant to be like an adventure with each day presenting a new opportunity to discover new things about life and yourself.

Your evolution is about expansion and exploration. How can you expand yourself and explore new horizons if you hang onto material objects? By doing so it is like attempting to keep the past current and you do not want to let it go. So thus you hang onto papers, books, and other physical objects that only serve to take up space.

If you truly desire to evolve yourself then it is essential for you to allow life to unfold organically and naturally each day. This means living in the moment and then letting go just as you do when you go see a good movie. After the movie you let it go and you are ready for a new adventure. You wouldn't want to keep seeing the same movie each day or each week would you? Life detox is about letting go and letting life present to you new adventures, new people and new places. This supports your evolution and will help to make you healthier as these new experiences will bring new feelings of excitement and joy to your heart.

Don't you think it is time that you give yourself a new holistic foundation to how you are going to live your life from now on? This life detox process is essential if you truly want to feel and look awesome and if you desire to reach your full potential.

Just as your car requires to get washed at times and you change the oil and filter and clean the spark plugs and such, so too does your life require cleansing and to be washed of things that are toxic and stifling to your well-being and evolution. How many years have you been holding on to material objects? How long have you been spending time with some people that you really do not enjoy being with, however, you do so just so you have someone to hang out with so you do not feel lonely.

Be honest with yourself my friend because as you do then you will see how you have created a life that is actually stifling to your growth and well-being. Look, people love hanging onto material objects, people and places because it gives them a feeling of belonging and a sense of worth.

Maybe now you can become conscious of the fact that you are doing these things to satisfy your need to be loved and to feel like you fit in. So now you can elevate your consciousness and seek to satisfy your need for love and fitting in by creating a holistic foundation that serves your expansion. This means you go out and make new friends.

You remove material objects that have been sitting for years and you do not need and you go out and purchase new items that will bring in new energy to your home.

Think of this as a spring cleaning for your entire life. This will serve to give you a holistic foundation that will continue to get you results in elevating your well-being and for your evolution.

So how do you go about this life detox process realistically and holistically? Well, you first sit down with yourself and begin to be honest with your feelings about the material objects, people and places that you are attached to. Simply ask yourself why do you have these things in your life? Is it because you really want them there or are they there because they satisfy one of your needs?

As you go through this list of people, places and objects you will begin to see how you have gotten attached to them. Now that your consciousness is elevated, you can choose to remove them from your life as to catapult your evolution and well-being.

You will be amazed at the shift you feel just by getting rid of material objects from your house. In fact, you will feel so much lighter by doing so. So, begin going through your house and removing the material objects and even clothes that you do not require or see any purpose for. Get 3 large boxes and label one as donations, one box label sale items which you will sell online or locally and the other box label trash.

So as you go through your house you simply pick out a material object that has been sitting around and you throw it into one of the 3 boxes. Pretty simple stuff, it only requires a consciousness shift and you can easily let go of material objects.

Also, people can be toxic to your life as well as they pull your frequency down when you hang out with them. I am sure you know how this feels. You have been with people that after spending time with them, you feel drained of energy. My friend, this is your clue to remove them from your life as they are pulling your health down. When you spend time with someone, you ought to be feel energized and happy. If you do not then it means that these people are not healthy for your evolution and health.

Again, simply go by how you feel with the people in your life. If you feel drained of energy from spending time with someone then let them go. You do not owe them an explanation as to why you are moving on other than saying you are changing your life and wanting to explore new horizons. This will remove a huge load from your life I assure you.

As I spoke about earlier, it is all about energy. The intention is to harmonize and elevate your energy levels. **You have to understand that everything in life is either uplifting your energy levels or it is pulling it down.**

So, you require becoming conscious of this fact and make every life decision based on how it will affect your energy levels. This is why doing a life detox can be the greatest blessing for you as it removes and purges all things that are pulling your frequency down. Your health levels are the direct result of how much energy you have pulsing through your body and how harmonized it is.

Begin to view life in terms of frequency and how everything in life is either elevating it or pulling it down. This means material objects, people and places. With each of these you will get a feeling and that feeling is your clue as to what effect it is having on your energy levels and frequency.

As you get more in tune with your body and begin to sense energies, this practice of observing how something is making you feel becomes natural.

By the way, as you clean up your body and nutrition and your life, you will be so connected and conscious that you will naturally choose the Higher choices in your life. This will translate into choosing better people to be friends with, you will enjoy being in nature more and you will simply be in the flow of life.

Your whole life will change obviously by going through this process so begin to expand your consciousness and allow it to happen. After all, this is why you are here on this planet, to express yourself and explore and expand your consciousness.

So my friend, begin to detox your life of all things that lower your frequency. Bring in new fresh energy with purchasing new clothes, new shoes, buy flowers and place them around your house and listen to new music. All of these things feed you with frequencies, so make sure they are holistic and harmonic in nature.

Nature is beautiful and is the direct link to your health and well-being. Begin to embody the holistic pathway I have set before you and you will see wonders before your eyes. This process can be a bit challenging because you will be surrendering things in your life that have become your safety zones. These things have put you inside a box, a paradigm if you will that are stifling to your evolution as a Sacred Being.

The pathway I have set before you is something that can continue to get you results. Essentially, you require embodying this life path and make it your number 1 priority as to do so will catapult your evolution and your health results. As you can see by now, my holistic slimming pathway has helped you to create a holistic foundation that can now serve you the rest of your life.

This is why almost all of the health and weight reduction programs that have come out in the past 20 years simply were not able to get most people lasting results. It is because they were and have been teaching erroneous philosophies and were only focusing on the physical aspect to health.

In actuality, everything is affecting your health my friend. Your job, your friends, your clothes, the music you listen to, the smell of your home, where you live, and even what kind of bed you sleep on are all affecting your health on some level. Once again, it is about energy and frequency. These aspects to your life will either elevate your energy or pull it down. Only you can know this.

Again, it is simply being in tune with your body and feeling how they make you feel. The feeling is your clue as to which they are doing. If you use this process of feeling in your life then you will make much Higher decisions consistently. It is kind of like when you go buy new shoes and you know the pair you buy is the one that feels the best. It just feels right. **Begin to feel your life and watch the elevation in your energy and your life experiences.**

Another area of your life that requires detoxing is the home cleaning products that you use to clean the house with. Become conscious of the fact that there are natural ways of doing things. Society has created many toxic compounds to do house chores that can easily be done with natural compounds.

Just so you know, is that these products are chemically based and can be quite toxic to your health. They are not required to clean your house with. The planet has had enough of the toxic chemicals my friend. One capful of laundry detergent will eventually contaminate hundreds of gallons of water as it goes through the water system.

These cleaning products are toxic and can be unhealthy for you to have them in your house as some may even outgas noxious fumes for many months. There are now plenty of natural alternatives to these toxic compounds.

I will gift you a super natural wonder cleaner. **You can use hydrogen peroxide to literally clean your entire house.** It is the greatest disinfectant and deodorizer on planet earth. You simply put it into a spray bottle and then you are set to clean. Spray it where you require it and let it sit for a few minutes. It will clean windows, mirrors, bathroom sinks, toilets, floors, counter tops, you can use it to clean your car with as in windows, mirrors, dashboard and even your tires. You can also use hydrogen peroxide to deodorize your house of any funky smells.

Simply put into a spray bottle and spray the air. You can also use it to disinfect any pet bowls, pet beds and anything else related to your pets. It can also be used to remove stains from clothes and carpets. Simply spray on the stain and let it sit for 30 minutes. For tougher stains keep spraying and rub the area for a few minutes and watch the beauty before your eyes.

Hydrogen peroxide can also be a great bug remover. If you ever have ants or any bugs in your house simply spray the area for a few minutes and the bugs are gone within seconds to minutes. Keep spraying the area for a few days if you have had an issue with ants or bugs for some time. They will not return after you do this. Do you see how nature can resolve many life issues and do it in a holistic manner.

The only thing required of you is to simply do it, use the natural stuff, walk your talk. Do not think about it, just do it for your own good and that of the planet.

Another natural compound that will help keep bugs away is diatomaceous earth powder. This compound is great as it will get rid of bugs fast and even roaches. Again, something natural to resolve a life issue that is holistic and safe and helps the planet be healthier as well.

Now that you are conscious of these facts it is up to you to simply embody them. I have gifted you 2 easy and low cost manners of helping you keep your house clean and bug free. What are you going to do with this knowledge now? Please step up to the plate and just follow what is being taught and you will see the benefits.

Another area of life that you require detoxing is your skin care products. Most skin care products have toxic ingredients in them and these can impact your health in negative ways. Begin to recycle your body care products with natural versions as they are a much better option for your health and well-being. Your body shall thank you.

I carry a super High Frequency line of body care products that are amazing. Please contact me to learn more about them.

Your affirmation for the week is:

I Now Release All Things That Are Toxic In My Life. I Easily Surrender These To Source and I Now Embrace New & Uplifting Experiences, People, and Places. I Love My New Life!

Week 11

Conscious Living

The Only Path For Maintaining Health and Wellness

- The Power of Your Consciousness and How To Use It For Creating A Victorious Life

- Your Consciousness and The Impact on The Entire Planet

- Conscious Living Expands Everyone and Everything

Ok, this is week 11 of your holistic makeover journey. Congratulations on making it this far! If you have followed what I have set before you in the previous 11 weeks then you are for sure doing so much better and have new experiences in your life. The pathway I have set before you is something that can continue to get you results. Essentially, you require embodying this life path and make it your number 1 priority as to do so will catapult your evolution and your health results.

As you learned by now, you are a multi-dimensional being and require caring for your full complex of mind, body and spirit. It is about being conscious and using your consciousness to create a life that is conducive to your well-being and evolution.

Most people think they are living consciously when in fact they are not. Simply observe the life of most people and you will see the disharmony, the drama, the low level health and the repeating of life patterns and cycles. These are all signs of unconsciousness and have become a normal thing in life for most people.

Unconsciousness is the result of wanting to cater to superficial desires and wants and putting the physical realm first.

You my friend are mainly a spiritual being and require honoring this Truth. Humanity has forgotten about its Sacred and Spiritual nature and has placed more importance on physical thrills and superficial gratification. Thus, you got what you have on this planet...unconsciousness. You can assist in the waking of humanity by cleaning up your entire life and being an example of what is possible for a human being.

You can at least be the catalyst to many people's awakening and evolution. This is the noblest gift you can give to humanity and Mother Earth. You can use your consciousness to change your life quite quickly. In fact, it is so simple that you miss it.

So, begin today using a Higher Conscious Awareness of how you live your life. Use your consciousness with every decision you make. Use your consciousness with every person you meet. Use your consciousness to expand your reality. You can do wonders if you simply maintain conscious awareness of what you are doing, what you are feeling, and what you are choosing in your life. Now go out there and rock your life and be an inspiration to others so we can finally purify this Sacred planet for health, happiness and peace.

Week 12

The Frequency Factor

This is going to be the most important lesson you learn out of the 12 week pathway I have set before you. So, ground yourself right now and listen very carefully. I am about to reveal to you some very powerful knowledge and wisdom that can profoundly elevate your life very quickly.

You see my friend, you are a very powerful being. If you truly knew just who you are and how powerful you are then you would be in complete joy and freedom. You are a co-creator with the Universe. You are creating your life every second of every day.

The issue is...you along with most of humanity have been conditioned and taught to use your power in a negative way. You are using your inner power of consciousness as to stifle yourself as opposed to enlighten and uplift yourself. Allow me to clarify.

In case you do not know, is that this Universe is designed in a vibrational way. Everything in the Universe is vibrating and pulsating a frequency...every star, planet, moon, solar system, galaxy...each one has its own unique frequency signature. Even colors, words and plants and animals have their own frequency signature as well.

You too my friend have your own unique frequency signature that you are blipping out to the Universe every second of every day. Some people may call this your vibe, call it what you like, however, you are a vibrating being, plain and simple.

Now, what you must comprehend is that the Universe is designed in nature that it is responding to your vibration to the exact level of what you are blipping out. Every belief you have, every opinion you have, every feeling you have about all topics of life are being mirrored to you in exact proportion to the degree of what you are resonating out to the Universe. This can be proven quite profoundly as the second you change your vibration, is when the Universe begins sending to you new life experiences, people and events.

In essence, the Universe is mirroring to you every single feeling you have about every topic of your life. The Universe is like a BIG magic genie and is always sending you what you are in essence blipping out to the Universe. Your feelings are very powerful and this is what the Universe is mainly listening to when it sends to you what you are resonating out. This is law my friend.

Some people in recent years have been talking about the Law of Attraction and such. Many of these teachings only have a few elements of the total piece of what the Law of Attraction really is and how it is literally bringing (attracting) to you as a magnet does...life events and people into your life.

Most of what you are blipping out to the Universe is unconscious so you are not aware of exactly what you are resonating out. However, if you want to truly know exactly what you are blipping out to the Universe then all you have to do is look at your life.

Look at the people and life patterns and such that keep showing up in your life. That is the quickest way for you to see what you are maintaining in your consciousness somewhere about any life topic.

Be aware that most of what you are blipping out is unconscious due to the fact that you have been conditioned and programmed by your family, school and society in general and you drew up conclusions when you were a child based on those philosophies, which many are limiting and some quite unhealthy.

Life doesn't just send you stuff. There is a vibration in your being that is magnetizing these events and people toward you. The Universe is simply mirroring to you what you are blipping out. The Universe is simply showing you what limiting and funny beliefs and attitudes you have about yourself and life and people. YOUR WISH IS YOUR COMMAND...is what the Universe is constantly delivering to you.

So, maybe now you will begin to use your consciousness with a little more awareness that you are co-creating your life with the Universe. I will now share with you a secret that can dramatically help catapult your life in quantum leaps.

The expression is **Change Your Frequency, Change Your Life**. As you begin to elevate your frequency, the Universe begins to send you new life events and new people as your Higher vibration is very attractive to the Universe.

Perhaps now you will comprehend why I have created my 12 week Holistic Lifestyle Makeover for you? I did so because it is one of the most effective ways to elevate your frequency as to help catapult your health and also your evolution. You must embody a holistic lifestyle if you are ever going to tap into your Higher Potentials and experience life on such a High level. **My 12 week pathway is literally a roadmap to your evolution as a human being**.

As you remove and vaporize unhealthy and limiting habits, people, places, nutrition choices, music, tv and more, you will automatically begin to see new experiences showing up in your life. **Life Is A Frequency Game!!!**

What you experience is directly attributed to your frequency and what you are blipping out to the Universe, it is this simple. My recommendation to you is...do everything you can to elevate your frequency as to do so will be a direct path to a Higher Life Experience.

Begin to incorporate more fun into your life and learn to embody a new feeling about life and yourself. Have more of a child like demeanor as you walk through life and you will see magic before your eyes. Learn to chill and relax and view life more as a game then something serious. View yourself as a great being that has value and is worthy of Prosperity, Happiness, Joy and Wellness.

Begin to embody these frequencies so the Universe can mirror them back to you. Be kinder, be gentler, be more loving, be happier, be more appreciative of who you are and what you have in your life. Be you in the greatest way possible. Show up in life 1,000,000 %.

Be EXTRAORDINARY, Be EXCEPTIONAL, STAND OUT & Be Unique in your own unique way. Share who you truly are with the world, it is ok, you now have permission to do so. I give you full approval to go out into the world and be the greatest you ever. Shine your light and your love with everyone.

Be you in the most amazing way possible and you will inspire many people in life. It is the greatest gift you can give yourself and humanity. Be the Angel Star you came to be. Spread your wings and fly so high that you touch the sky.

Express your True Self and share your Truth with everyone as to do so will help them to share their Truth with you. Seek to ignite the potential in others with your kind words and smile.

You just never know what you may ignite in others by you simply being you and being an inspiration to them. As you learn to play this game of life with the Higher Frequencies, you will be the catalyst to many people's evolution.

On this glorious day, you are granted the freedom to be YOU in all your glory and in your FULL POTENTIAL. You are hereby granted permission and approval to express, to explore and to inspire yourself and humanity for the greater good of all. Now go out and rock your life sweet angel star!!! Humanity is waiting...

I wish you many blessings on your High Flying Journey!!!

To Your Victorious Life,

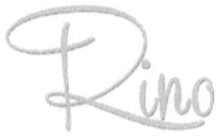

Rino Soriano is known as the **Conscious Health Alchemist** and is a Intuitive Holistic Health Coach and Holistic Lifestyle Coach.

Rino offers personalized coaching programs for people wanting to get fit, get slim, get healthy, get energized, get cleansed, or experience life on a Higher level and who want to rock their life. Please visit his website for more information on his coaching programs. **RinoSoriano.com**

You can visit Rino's Holistic Store to view and learn more about health resources and tools that can assist you on your makeover journey.

Rino's other life transforming books:

Body Brilliance, The 8 Royal Diamonds For A Healthier and More Radiant You

Youngevity Revolution, The 12 Secret Spirals of Enduring Youth and Longevity

Fun Food Fantastic, Knock Your Socks Off Meal Creations

Mystic Smoothies, The 33 Most Nutritious and Delicious Smoothies To Rock The Planet

Consciousity, The Crystalline Key For Transforming Earth Blue

Bodybuilding Brilliance, Massive Muscle Makeover

Flying Hawk Productions